SECOND EDITION

A PRACTICAL APPROACH TO
ANALYZING
HEALTHCARE
DATA

SUSAN WHITE, PHD, CHDA

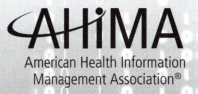

American Health Information
Management Association®

ISBN: **978-1-58426-421-7**
AHIMA Product No.: AC216113

AHIMA Staff:
Jessica Block, MA, Assistant Editor
Katherine M. Greenock, MS, Production Development Editor
Jason O. Malley, Director, Creative Content Development
Pamela Woolf, Managing Editor

The websites listed in this book were current and valid as of the date of publication. However, webpage addresses and the information on them may change at any time. The user is encouraged to perform his or her own general web searches to locate any site addresses listed here that are no longer valid.

CPT® is a registered trademark of the American Medical Association. CHDA® is a registered trademark of the American Health Information Management Association. All other copyrights and trademarks mentioned in this book are the possession of their respective owners. AHIMA makes no claim of ownership by mentioning products that contain such marks.

For more information, including updates, about AHIMA Press publications, visit http://www.ahima.org/publications/updates.aspx

American Health Information Management Association
233 North Michigan Avenue, 21st Floor
Chicago, Illinois 60601-5809
ahima.org

Contents

About the Author

Susan White, PhD, CHDA, is an Associate Professor of Clinical Health and Rehabilitation Sciences in the Health Information Management and Systems Division at The Ohio State University. Dr. White teaches classes in statistics, data analytics, healthcare finance, and computer applications. She has written numerous books regarding the benchmarking of healthcare facilities and appropriate use of claims data. She has also published articles covering outcomes assessment and risk adjustment using healthcare financial and clinical data analysis, hospital benchmarking, predictive modeling, and claims data mining. Prior to joining OSU, Dr. White was a Vice President for Research and Development for both Cleverley & Associates and CHIPS/Ingenix. She has 15 years of experience in the practice of healthcare financial and revenue cycle consulting in addition to her academic experience.

Acknowledgments

I would like to acknowledge Lynn Kuehn for all of the hard work she did in writing the first edition of this text. I am thankful to have the opportunity to expand on her work and follow her lead in balancing the technical and practical aspects of data analysis. I would also like to thank Dr. Melanie Brodnik, the HIMS Division Director at OSU. She provided endless mentoring and advice on this and many other projects. I also would like to thank my family for their indulgence while I spent many an evening and weekend writing this text.

Foreword

Welcome to the second edition of *A Practical Approach to Analyzing Healthcare Data*. Susan White, PhD, CHDA, the author of this edition, has taken the discussion in the first edition to the next level.

When the first edition was written, HIM professionals were beginning to flourish in the data analyst role. Many HIM professionals performed data analysis in their roles but may not have thought of it as data analysis. Therefore, *A Practical Approach to Analyzing Healthcare Data* was written to help these professional improve their analysis skills and also help prepare candidates for the certified health data analyst (CHDA) examination, which had just been launched. However, with the evolving role of HIM professionals in data analytics, a more comprehensive but still practical treatment of the subject is now required. The industry is moving and is in need of this new, enhanced second edition.

The easy readability of the first edition has been maintained while strengthening the statistical foundation of HIM data analytics. The second edition works equally well for professional development and classroom use. The expansion of the statistical chapters will assist learning in the classroom setting. The examples continue to be based in real life HIM scenarios. Instructors will find a complete complement of instructor resources in the downloadable, online resources.

The first three chapters set the stage for learning with an introduction to data analysis, a description of types of healthcare data, and a discussion of tools used in data analysis. The statistical chapters, 4 through 6, have been greatly enhanced and reorganized into a discussion of categorical variables, continuous variables, and the relationships between two or more variables. These chapters are now structured to describe each technique and its mechanics, along with an interpretation and example for each technique. Formulas are displayed, along with their associated results, for many of the data analysis projects performed in the HIM field.

Chapter 7 guides the learner through the sample selection process. And a new chapter (8) on exploratory data applications covers HIM data examples in a variety of types of DRG systems, the APC system, utilization patterns, and RVU data. Chapter 9 discusses benchmarking and analyzing externally reported data.

The appendices provide information about the downloadable resources accompanying the book including a glossary, selected data analyst biographies and job descriptions, and information on AHIMA's CHDA credential.

This second edition provides HIM professionals and students with an excellent resource for their journey in understanding healthcare data and data analytics. Enjoy this enhanced treatment of healthcare analytics.

—Lynn Kuehn, MS, RHIA, CCS-P, FAHIMA
Author of the first edition of *A Practical Approach to Analyzing Healthcare Data*

Introduction

Data analysis is a growing area for health information management (HIM) professionals as the field further evolves from gathering data to managing information. The role of the data analyst is to acquire, manage, manipulate, and analyze data and then report the results. Knowledge in this area has previously been obtained through experience and experimentation. In addition, *A Practical Approach to Analyzing Healthcare Data* was written to help professionals learn analysis skills in an organized fashion and fill the role of data analyst effectively.

> As stated in *Vision 2016: A Blueprint for Quality Education in Health Information Management*: It is expected in the future that we will need experts to process and edit coded data, not to actually code the data. In 2016, it will still be important to teach "how to code," but it will be more important to teach critical thinking skills that focus on the analysis and reporting of data sets and greater assurance of quality data (AHIMA 2007, 7).

Additionally, *Vision 2016* encourages entry-level students to specialize in coding as a track to serve as a basis for more advanced education in data analysis. At the same time, *Vision 2016* presents educators with a challenge to implement more critical thinking skills on data analysis into the curriculum.

To help answer that challenge, this book provides critical thinking exercises in the following areas:

- Assess data needs, design data collection process, coordinate data collection, collect data, interpret data, and report information
- Analyze and present data for quality management, utilization management, risk management, and other patient care-related studies
- Provide data for healthcare decision making such as quality, safety, and effectiveness of healthcare

Curriculum knowledge clusters that are addressed in the text are:

IA 5   Secondary data sources (registries and indexes; databases—such as MEDPAR, NPDB, HCUP) (4)

IC 2   Medicare Severity Diagnosis Related Groups (MS-DRGs) (4)

IIA 1   Statistical analysis on healthcare data (5)

IIA 2   Descriptive statistics (such as means, standard deviations, frequencies, ranges, percentiles) (5)

IIA 6   Data reporting and presentation techniques (5)

IIA 8   Research design and methods (such as quantitative, qualitative, evaluative, outcomes) (5)

IIB 2   Utilization and resource management (4)

The concepts of acquiring, managing, manipulating, and analyzing data are the core material of this book. This book assumes that the reader has a solid knowledge of how codes are assigned to diagnoses and procedures using the ICD-9-CM and CPT and HCPCS coding systems in both the hospital and physician setting and does not teach the concepts of coding. Other texts and distance education classes are available from AHIMA to teach coding using both of these systems. If the reader does not have a solid knowledge base, prerequisite or concurrent study in these areas is recommended.

In addition, readers are expected to have a working knowledge of basic statistics and statistical formulae, as well as an intermediate knowledge of Microsoft Office Excel for data entry, creating formulas, and creating presentation graphs. Prerequisite or concurrent study in these areas is also recommended.

It should be noted that discussions of Excel, SAS, and SPSS software do not imply endorsement of these products, only that they are commonly used within the field of data analytics.

This book is focused on real-life data problem solving. Whenever possible, readers are provided with real data or asked to research real data using the Internet resources publicly available.

Introduction to Data Analysis

Data Analysis

Healthcare is a data driven business. **Data** is collected regarding diagnostic tests and treatment delivered to patients. Providers give surveys to patients to determine their level of satisfaction. Data is transmitted from providers to payers to determine the proper payment for services. The implementation of electronic health records (EHRs) is expanding the amount of data available for analysis exponentially. These sources of data have a primary purpose of delivering and measuring healthcare services. The data may also serve a secondary purpose of benchmarking providers or determining the most efficient way to deliver healthcare services.

Data analysis is primarily defined as the task of transforming, summarizing, or modeling data to allow the user to make meaningful conclusions. Data analysis may be characterized as turning data into information that may be used for operational decision making. Data analysts bring meaning to a table of values that would otherwise be overwhelming. The healthcare industry uses information gathered from data analysis to measure the quality of care and the efficiency of care delivery.

When data is analyzed to make conclusions regarding the primary reason for the data collection, the analysis is referred to as **primary data analysis**. The use of data for other purposes is considered **secondary data analysis**. For example, following the trend in a patient's blood glucose level over time to diagnose diabetes is an example of primary data analysis. The primary purpose of collecting blood glucose level is for diagnosis of a disease. The timing of postoperative blood glucose levels for cardiac surgery patients may also be used as a quality indicator (AHRQ 2012). This is an example of a secondary use. While the primary use of blood glucose levels inform the provider about the patient's condition, the timing of the collection can be analyzed to inform the provider about the postsurgical monitoring process, and thus, is secondary data analysis. Using billing and coding data to determine payment for services is also a **primary use** of data. Analyzing billing data to benchmark cost or utilization statistics is a **secondary use**. When using data for secondary analysis, the analyst must always be aware of the primary use to ensure the data collection method and content is appropriate for the secondary analysis.

Data analysis may be segmented into two broad categories: descriptive and inferential statistics. **Descriptive statistics** literally describe the **distribution** of the data. The distribution of the data is characterized by the center, or typical value, and the spread, or variation observed in the data. The typical value may be described using statistics such as the mean, median, or mode of the data. The variance, or spread of the values of the data, may be measured using variance, standard deviation, or range of the values.

It is not possible or practical for a data analyst to observe the values of a variable in the entire population of interest. Instead, many studies are based on a sample or subset of the population. For example, an HIM director may want to study the coding accuracy of contract coding staff. It is not feasible to recode every chart to measure the accuracy rate in the population of all charts coded by the contract staff, but a random sample may be selected and recoded. The results of that sample audit may then be used to make conclusions about the population using inferential statistics.

Qualitative Versus Quantitative Analysis

Healthcare data may be assigned to two broad categories: qualitative and quantitative. Understanding the differences between these two categories will help a data analyst choose the appropriate approach for analyzing and reporting data.

Qualitative data describes observations about a subject. For instance, a nurse may observe that a patient is disoriented and note that in the health record. The concept of disoriented cannot be measured numerically, but can be coded using either International Classification of Diseases, ninth revision, Clinical Modification (ICD-9-CM), International Classification of Diseases, tenth revision, Clinical Modification (ICD-10-CM), or Systemized Nomenclature of Medicine (SNOMED) coding. The frequency of the assigned codes or even the frequency of the key term disoriented may be summarized. It would not make sense to try to take the average of disorientation, but it would be useful to know what percent of the patients present with that symptom. Open-ended responses to surveys are another example of qualitative data. Responses to questions such as: "How could we make your stay more pleasant?," "What is your favorite color?" or "What is your occupation?" are not naturally numeric, but can be recoded to allow the frequency of similar responses to be summarized.

Qualitative data can be categorized and summarized, but they are not naturally numeric values. The categorized qualitative data may take two forms:

1. **Nominal scale** data – discrete categories with no inferred order; examples of nominal data include diagnosis codes, procedure codes, color, clinical units.
2. **Ordinal scale** data – discrete categories with a natural or inferred order; examples of ordinal data include patient satisfaction responses on a five-point scale, patient severity scores.

Quantitative data is naturally numeric. Qualitative observations may be confirmed using quantitative data. For instance, a patient may feel abnormally hot to the touch. That qualitative observation can be confirmed by taking the patient's temperature and recording the value in the health record. Quantitative data may also be categorized into two forms:

1. **Interval scale** data – Numeric data where the distance between two values has meaning, but multiplying values has no meaning. Temperature measurement is an example of interval data. 30 degrees Celsius is 10 degrees warmer than 20; and 40 degrees is 10 degrees warmer than 30, but 40 degrees is not twice as warm as 20 degrees. The value of zero has no interpretation in interval data scales. Again, temperature is a good example; zero degrees is very cold, but it is not the absence of temperature.
2. **Ratio scale** data – Number data where zero has an interpretation and the values may be doubled or multiplied by a constant and still have meaning. Examples of ratio data include: currency, length of stay, number of admissions, and age.

Quantitative data can be either discrete or continuous. Discrete data includes a finite number of values. There are spaces between values on a number line. Counting data is typically discrete in nature; for example, one-half of an admission does not have meaning. In contrast, continuous data can take on fractional and whole number values.

David Bowers presents an excellent decision tree for determining the measurement scale of data (2008). Figure 1.1 is adapted to use the terminology consistent with this text.

Figure 1.1 Variable scale decision tree

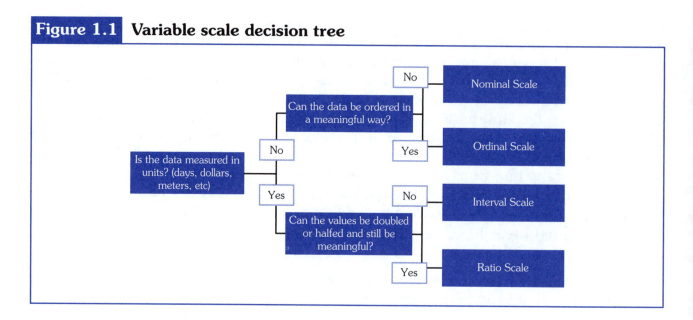

Types of Analysis

The first step in any data analysis exercise is determining the type of data to be analyzed: categorized qualitative (nominal or ordinal) or quantitative (interval or ratio). The analyst may then make an informed decision regarding the descriptive or inferential statistical techniques to be used. Data available to be analyzed are typically collected by sampling from a population of subjects of interest. The concepts of sample and population are covered in depth in chapter 7.

Descriptive Statistics

Descriptive statistics are used to summarize the center and shape of the distribution of a variable of interest. The **variable** of interest is an attribute or quantity that is the focus of an analysis. Two attributes of the data are most important to end users: "What is the typical value?" and "How spread out are the values?" If the data is qualitative, then the categorization or recoding of the data may be necessary prior to summarizing.

Calculating descriptive statistics is the first step in a data analysis project. These statistics are found throughout healthcare. CMS uses the mean and median cost of services to set payment rates for the hospital inpatient and outpatient prospective payment systems. The use of descriptive statistics applied to actual claims experience ensures that the payment rates are calibrated to reflect the relative resource intensity of providing services to Medicare beneficiaries. The mean and median are examples of measures of central tendency or the center of a distribution that may be used with data measured on a continuous scale (interval or ratio). The calculation of the mean and median is presented in chapter 5.

In addition to measuring the typical value or center of a distribution of a data set, descriptive statistics may also be used to measure the spread of the data values. Common measures of spread include the variance and standard deviation. The range of values may also be reported to describe the spread of the distribution.

Categorical or discrete values such as those measured on nominal and ordinal scales may be described using the mode, or most frequent value. Proportions or percentages of values by category may also be reported for discrete data. Qualitative data, once coded, may also be described using the mode or proportions.

Table 1.1 presents the four basic data scales and the most commonly used descriptive statistics for each scale. Recall that the first step in determining which descriptive statistic to apply to a data set is to determine the measurement scale or data type. For instance, favorite color is a nominal scale data element. Taking the mean or average favorite color of a group does not make sense. Similarly, calculating the mode for the charges incurred by a sample of patients would not be meaningful, as it is unlikely that any patients would have exactly the same charges. If they did, there is no guarantee that they would be in the center of the distribution. The mode does not provide useful information about the typical value of a continuous variable.

Table 1.1 Data types and descriptive statistics

Data Type	Definition	Examples	Appropriate Descriptive Statistics
Nominal	Categorical data where the categories are mutually exclusive, but do not have a natural order.	Gender, HCPCS codes, department or unit	Frequency counts, proportions, mode
Ordinal	Categorical data where the categories are mutually exclusive and they do have a natural order.	Patient satisfaction scores, severity scores, trauma center level, surveys measured on a Likert scale	Frequency counts, proportions, mode, range
Interval	Naturally numeric data where the distance between two values has meaning, but multiplying values and zero value has no interpretation.	Temperature, pH level	Mean, median, standard deviation, range
Ratio	Naturally numeric data where zero has an interpretation and the values may be doubled or multiplied by a constant and still have meaning.	Charges, length of stay or age	Mean, median, standard deviation, range, geometric mean, coefficient of variation

Source: AHIMA Press. LaTour 2012.

Statistics such as readmission rates, mortality rates, average cost, and average length of stay are all found in management reports. These quantities are considered descriptive statistics and are commonly used throughout healthcare. A hospital's case mix index (CMI) is an example of a descriptive statistic that is frequently used. The CMI is the average or mean relative weight of the diagnosis-related group (DRG) assigned to a hospital's discharges. The CMI is sometimes used as a proxy for the severity of patients treated by a hospital. A higher weighted DRG is indicative of an admission that requires a higher level of resource intensity and is assigned a higher payment. Averaging the DRG relative weight for all patients discharged describes the typical resource intensity of the patients treated at a hospital.

Inferential Statistics

Inferential statistics is the set of techniques that are used to make conclusions about the population of interest based on the analysis of a sample of the data. Common inferential statistic techniques include the use of confidence intervals and hypothesis testing. A **confidence interval** is a range calculated based on a sample that is likely to include the true population value of a parameter. If an analyst wishes to estimate the average length of stay at a hospital based on a sample of patients, a confidence interval provides a range of values for which he can be 90 percent or 95 percent sure the population length of stay is included. Confidence intervals are often reported for opinion surveys. A survey of patient satisfaction may result in 90 percent plus or minus two percent of the patients agreeing that the care they received was good to excellent. The plus or minus two percent represents the width of the confidence interval for the overall satisfaction (88 percent to 92 percent).

   Hypothesis testing allows an analyst to measure the strength of evidence from the data to reject or not reject a hypothesis. Typically, rejecting a hypothesis requires some action to be taken or cost to be incurred, so the analyst would like the probability of making an incorrect conclusion based on the data to be small (less than five percent). Hypothesis testing allows the analyst to make decisions and measure the probability of making an error. Statistical hypotheses are tested using a test statistic that typically compares what we would expect to occur under a null hypothesis to what we observe in the sampled data.

   Inferential statistics are reported by the **Centers for Medicare and Medicaid Services (CMS)** on their **Hospital Compare** website (see online Appendix G). Figure 1.2 is an example of using confidence intervals to compare a facility's mortality rate to a standard. In this example, the standard is the national death rate for heart attack patients (15.5 percent). The standard is represented by the dotted vertical line in each facility's bar. The facility's rate is displayed on their bar. For instance, the death rate for heart attack patients at Riverside Methodist Hospital is 17.7 percent. The shaded interval represents a confidence interval around the facility-specific death rate. If the shaded interval includes the national rate, then we conclude that the facility's rate is not statistically different than the standard or national death rate. The width of the confidence interval shows the precision of the estimate of the death rate. A narrower interval is more precise; a wider interval is less precise.

Exploratory Data Analysis and Data Mining

Exploratory data analysis (EDA) and **data mining** are both used to uncover patterns in data. The two terms are often used interchangeably in practice. EDA traditionally uses graphical techniques to display the data and identify outliers or trends. With the introduction of larger datasets in healthcare, the term data mining is gaining more

Figure 1.2 **Hospital Compare example**

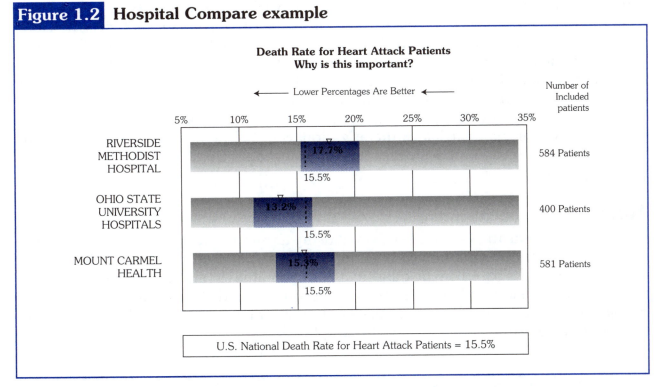

Death Rate for Heart Attack Patients
Why is this important?

◄—— Lower Percentages Are Better ◄——

Number of
Included
patients

	RIVERSIDE METHODIST HOSPITAL	17.7% / 15.5%	584 Patients
	OHIO STATE UNIVERSITY HOSPITALS	13.2% / 15.5%	400 Patients
	MOUNT CARMEL HEALTH	15.3% / 15.5%	581 Patients

U.S. National Death Rate for Heart Attack Patients = 15.5%

Source: Center for Medicare and Medicaid Services Hospital Compare, 2012.

popularity for this activity. Data mining uses both graphical techniques and descriptive statistics to identify trends and patterns in data.

Data mining may be used in healthcare to identify high or low performing providers and to determine subsets of the population that may be using significant portions of healthcare resources. Data mining may also be used to identify opportunities to improve the financial performance of a healthcare provider. For instance, the techniques may be used to identify services that are denied most often by a particular payer or diagnosis codes that are most often missed as complications or comorbidities.

Predictive Modeling

In **predictive modeling**, the analyst uses historical data to find trends or patterns in the data that can then help predict future outcomes. Data mining is often used to identify the best predictors of future performance. Statistical models, such as regression or cluster analysis, are used to formulate models that determine the most likely outcome. For example, an analyst may determine that they can accurately predict the length of stay for a patient based on their reason for admission, age, and procedure to be performed during the admission. If a patient's length of stay goes beyond the predicted value, then that case may be given extra scrutiny by the utilization management team to determine if the longer stay is necessary.

CMS currently uses predictive modeling to identify fraudulent claims prior to payment (White 2011). Predictive models are used to determine the likelihood that a claim is fraudulent. If a claim is determined to have a high probability of representing a claim either submitted in error or through deliberate fraudulent activity, the claim may be reviewed prior to payment. The models may use data elements specific to both the provider and the patient. For example, a claim for an appendectomy may be flagged for further review if the patient had an appendectomy on a previous claim. Provider demographic data may be used to identify claims that are outside the scope of service previously provided by that provider. For instance, an orthopedic surgeon is unlikely to submit a claim for a cardiac catheterization. Such a claim would be identified and reviewed to ensure it is an accurate reporting of the services provided to the patient prior to payment.

Auditing

Health record **auditing** is often performed using a random sample of records. The size of that sample and the method of selection are both based on statistical analysis. The size of the sample is based on the quantity to be estimated (a rate or a payment amount), the desired precision and confidence of the estimate, and the sampling technique to be used. Once those questions are answered, inferential statistical techniques may be employed to determine the appropriate sample size.

Skills Required for Data Analysis

Qualitative analysis requires inductive reasoning skills and can be more subjective than quantitative analysis. This type of analysis is best completed by someone who is inquisitive and might wonder whether one occurrence in the data means that it could be a wider problem. Quantitative analysis involves deductive reasoning skills and can be more objective because work is done on rates, frequencies of events, totals, and percentages.

In addition to these general abilities, analysis of coded data requires that the analyst have a solid knowledge of how codes are assigned in the area that is being analyzed. Data analysis is not typically performed by a novice coder or without the assistance of a coder with advanced knowledge.

Data analysts often combine knowledge of coded data with general health information management (HIM) knowledge about the structure of data and a working knowledge of information technology such as database structures and common software packages. Data analysts working in organizations that have EHRs also need a working knowledge of the EHR structure and the data elements collected in the EHR.

The following skills are also helpful to the effective analyst:

- Development and implementation of data collection systems and other strategies
- Design of small-scale databases and use of relational databases
- Use of a statistical software package for analyzing large data sets
- Use of various query tools
- Ability to see potential relationships between data elements

- Ability to present complex information in an understandable and compelling manner
- Critical thinking skills
- Project management skills

Opportunities for Health Information Management Professionals in Healthcare Data Analytics

HIM professionals are uniquely positioned to take on a variety of roles related to healthcare data analytics. Combining the following skills transforms the traditional HIM role into one of a business analyst:

- Understand data structures and coding systems
- Understand available data and methods for integration
- Can communicate with both finance and IT staff
- Act as a business analyst—far more valuable than a pure data analyst

For instance, in revenue cycle management, the identification of missed charges is challenging. The traditional approach to identifying missed charges is to perform a charge description master (CDM) review and interview unit staff to ensure charge codes are utilized as designed. The staff may also review departmental order sheets to ensure they include complete and accurate listings of the services available in the department. An HIM professional with strong analytic skills may take a data-driven approach to identify cases with potential missed charges.

The charge codes that occur together often may be identified through profiling of the historical claims data. Claims with only one of those codes may be selected for focused review. A record review on that subset of records identified as likely to include missed charges may then be completed to understand the root cause of the missing charges. The use of analytics on the historical claims may save a significant amount of time in the identification of particular codes that are problematic. Corrective action may be designed and implemented in a much more efficient manner.

Opportunities to apply analytics to common operational issues are present throughout the healthcare business setting. AHIMA's Healthcare Data Analysis Toolkit lists a number of responsibilities that may be required of HIM professionals to perform analysis-based jobs in healthcare (Bronnert et al. 2011).

An entry-level health data analyst position may include the following analytic responsibilities:

- Identify, analyze, and interpret trends or patterns in complex data sets
- In collaboration with others, interpret data and develop recommendations on the basis of findings
- Develop graphs, reports, and presentations of project results, trends, data mining
- Perform basic statistical analyses for projects and reports

- Create and present quality dashboards
- Generate routine and ad hoc reports

A mid-level health data analyst position may include the following additional analytic responsibilities:

- Work collaboratively with data and reporting and the database administrator to help produce effective production management and utilization management reports in support of performance management related to utilization, cost, and risk with the various health plan data; monitor data integrity and quality of reports on a monthly basis
- Work collaboratively with data and reporting in monitoring financial performance in each health plan
- Develop and maintain claims audit reporting and processes
- Develop and maintain contract models in support of contract negotiations with health plans
- Develop, implement, and enhance evaluation and measurement models for the quality, data and reporting, and data warehouse department programs, projects, and initiatives for maximum effectiveness
- Recommend improvements to processes, programs, and initiatives by using analytical skills and a variety of reporting tools
- Determine the most appropriate approach for internal and external report design, production, and distribution, specific to the relevant audience

A senior-level health data analyst position may include the following additional analytic responsibilities:

- Understand and address the information needs of governance, leadership, and staff to support continuous improvement of patient care processes and outcomes
- Lead and manage efforts to enhance the strategic use of data and analytic tools to improve clinical care processes and outcomes continuously
- Work to ensure the dissemination of accurate, reliable, timely, accessible, actionable information (data analysis) to help leaders and staff actively identify and address opportunities to improve patient care and related processes
- Work actively with information technology to select and develop tools to enable facility governance and leadership to monitor the progress of quality, patient safety, service, and related metrics continuously throughout the system
- Engage and collaborate with information technology and senior leadership to create and maintain a succinct report (e.g., dashboard), as well as a balanced set of system assessment measures, that conveys status and direction of key system-wide quality and patient safety initiatives for the trustee quality and safety committee and senior management; present this information regularly to the quality and safety committee of the board to ensure understanding of information contained therein

- Actively support the efforts of divisions, departments, programs, and clinical units to identify, obtain, and actively use quantitative information needed to support clinical quality monitoring and improvement activities
- Function as an advisor and technical resource regarding the use of data in clinical quality improvement activities
- Lead analysis of outcomes and resource utilization for specific patient populations as necessary
- Lead efforts to implement state-of-the-art quality improvement analytical tools (i.e., statistical process control)
- Play an active role, including leadership, where appropriate, on teams addressing system-wide clinical quality improvement opportunities

The level of understanding of the relationship between variables analyzed and the complexity of the analytic techniques increase as an HIM professional advances from the entry to senior level. The common thread through all of these job responsibilities is strong basic analytic skills and understanding of the healthcare application of those techniques. HIM professionals that have a solid grasp of statistical techniques can combine those skills with their knowledge of the clinical application of data to assist with the interpretation and application of the results of analysis projects.

 Review Questions

1. Which of the following is the primary use of healthcare claims data?
   a. Analysis of utilization of healthcare resources
   b. Measurement of severity of illness
   c. Calculation of reimbursement for services
   d. Measurement of patient satisfaction

2. Which of the following data are categorized as ordinal?
   a. Favorite color
   b. Patient severity
   c. ICD-9-CM diagnosis codes
   d. Physician specialty

3. Data collected in response to the following prompt would be characterized as what type of data: "Please list any suggestions for improvement in your experience as a patient in our facility:"
   a. Interval
   b. Ratio
   c. Qualitative
   d. Quantitative

4. Which data type does not have a natural order?
   a. Ordinal
   b. Ratio
   c. Nominal
   d. Interval

5. Statistical methods that are used to find patterns in data are characterized as:
   a. Inferential statistics
   b. Auditing
   c. Exploratory data analysis
   d. Predictive modeling

6. Predictive modeling:
   a. Uses historical data to help determine future outcomes
   b. Describes the distribution of the data
   c. Finds patterns in data
   d. Allows decision making based on data

7. Which of the following are considered descriptive statistics?
   a. Mean
   b. Standard deviation
   c. Range
   d. All of the above

8. A hypothesis test is an example of:
   a. Descriptive statistics
   b. Inferential statistics
   c. A measurement of spread
   d. Data mining

9. The mean is an appropriate measure of the center of the distribution for which of the following variables?
   a. Evaluation and management level
   b. Patient severity
   c. Length of stay
   d. Mortality

10. The relative value unit (RVU) associated with a Current Procedural Terminology (CPT) code is an example of which variable type?
    a. Ordinal
    b. Nominal
    c. Interval
    d. Ratio

📖 References

Agency for Healthcare Research and Quality (AHRQ). 2012. Surgical Care Improvement Project: Percent of Cardiac Surgery Patients with Controlled 6 A.M. Postoperative Blood Glucose. http://qualitymeasures.ahrq.gov/content.aspx?id=35532

Bronnert, J., Clark, J., Hyde, L., Solberg, J., White, S., Wolin, M. 2011. *Health Data Analysis Toolkit*. Chicago: AHIMA.

Bowers. 2008. *Medical Statistics from Scratch*, 2nd ed. West Sussex, England: John Wiley & Sons.

LaTour, E. M. 2012. *Information Management: Concepts, Principles and Practice*, 4th ed. Chicago: AHIMA.

White, S. 2011. Predictive Modeling 101. *AHIMA* 82(9): 46–47.

Data in Healthcare

KEY TERMS

Ambulatory payment classification

CMS-1500

Current Procedural Terminology

Diagnostic data

Diagnosis-related group

Healthcare Common Procedure Coding System

Inpatient prospective payment system

Logical Observation Identifiers Names and Codes

Major diagnostic category

National Drug Codes

Outpatient Prospective Payment System

Procedural data

Relative value unit

Remittance advice

Revenue code

Uniform Bill-04 (UB-04)

Unstructured data

Types of Healthcare Data

It is imperative for data analysts to know where to locate both internal and external data of different types that may be useful during the analysis process. Today's healthcare data come from a variety of sources such as electronic health records, patient care systems, monitoring instruments, tracking registries, patient satisfaction surveys, and quality indictor surveys, as well as traditional coded data. While most of this data is generated from within the organization, other data may be obtained from external sources, such as through health information exchanges, or from the patient. Together all of this data creates a collection of information that seems to grow continuously. This chapter will discuss various types of data, from coded to administrative to registry data, that are available for analysis in healthcare today. It will also discuss the sources of comparative data available within the industry.

Multiple coding systems are used to describe healthcare services and the diagnoses for which those services are provided. Much of healthcare data is coded using industry-standard systems so the data can be aggregated, analyzed, and compared. These codes are used for reimbursement or for data submission to an external organization. The various types of data commonly found in healthcare are summarized below.

Diagnostic Data

Diagnostic data is the data obtained when diagnoses or reasons for visit are coded with a diagnostic classification system. All United States healthcare settings currently use the International Classification of Diseases, ninth revision, Clinical Modification, or ICD-9-CM, diagnosis codes to describe diagnoses or the reasons for the provision of healthcare services. This system has been in use since January 1, 1979, and is tentatively scheduled for replacement on October 1, 2014, with the Internal Classification of Diseases, tenth revision, Clinical Modification, or ICD-10-CM. The 10th revision provides thousands more codes with increased specificity. It also features a complete, standard description for each individual code, rather than a partial descriptor, as found in the current system.

As part of the **inpatient prospective payment system (IPPS)**, the Centers for Medicare and Medicaid Services (CMS) uses two code groupings to organize data and process payment. ICD-9-CM codes are used to compute the **diagnosis-related group**, or **DRG**, for each inpatient discharge. Each of these DRGs falls within a larger grouping, known as a **major diagnostic category**, or **MDC**; MDCs group similar DRGs together. DRGs and MDCs are not coded. They are computed using a DRG grouper program based on patient demographic data and the coded data that has been assigned to an inpatient case.

CMS changed the methodology for DRG grouping in October 2007. Prior to October 1, 2007, CMS grouped discharges using the original DRG system, which had been in place since 1982 and was commonly referred to as CMS-DRGs. As of October 1, 2007, CMS now groups and pays for inpatient care based on the Medicare severity-adjusted DRG, or MS-DRG, system. The MS-DRG system continues to use MDCs as an additional grouping methodology.

The complete listing of all MS-DRGs and their associated data (including the MDC assignment) is found as Table_5_IPPS_Final_Rule_for_FY13.xlsx as part of the online resources that accompany this book. This file can be found annually in the IPPS Final Rule published by CMS.

Procedural Data

Procedural data is the data obtained when procedures are coded using a procedural classification system. The ICD-9-CM system, for example, contains a procedural coding system that is used to code procedures performed on hospital inpatients. This system is being replaced in 2014 with the ICD-10-PCS, or ICD-10 Procedure Coding System, and will be required for use only for coding and reporting of hospital inpatient procedures.

Hospital outpatient services and all Medicare Part B services are coded with and will continue to be coded with the **CPT**, or **Current Procedural Terminology**, system developed to describe physician services and maintained by the American Medical Association.

CMS maintains a coding system that supplements CPT called the **Healthcare Common Procedure Coding System**, or **HCPCS**. HCPCS codes have five digits, starting with an alphabetic character. This system provides codes to be used specifically for Medicare beneficiaries and codes for drugs and supplies for submission to any payer. Drug codes begin with the letter J and describe a specific drug and dose. These are not specific to the manufacturer or generic versus brand status. HCPCS J codes are used to code drugs on physician and hospital outpatient claims (Kuehn 2013, 135).

The **Outpatient Prospective Payment System (OPPS)** uses a grouping methodology called **ambulatory payment classification** groups, or **APC**s, to group hospital outpatient services that use similar amounts and types of resources. APCs are not coded; they are computed based on the CPT or HCPCS codes assigned to the outpatient case.

The complete listing of all APCs and their associated data (including the relative weight and payment rates) is found as Addendum_C_HOPPS_Final_Rule_FY13.xlsx as part of the online resources that accompany this book. This file can be found annually in the Final Rule for the hospital outpatient prospective system (HOPPS) published by CMS.

Pharmacy Data

Hospital and retail pharmacies use **National Drug Codes**, or **NDC**s, to describe drugs. NDCs indicate the size of the package, the dosage formulation of the drug, the drug name (generic versus brand name), and the manufacturer. The codes are standardized by the National Council on Prescription Drugs Program (NCPDP). These 11-digit codes are found in the pharmacy file and are coded as the prescription is ordered. Digits one through five describe the manufacturer, digits six through nine describe the drug name, and digits 10 and 11 describe the package size and type. The NDC database is available on the FDA website (see online appendix G).

While specificity of NDC codes provides detailed information about the drugs used in a facility, this can make data analysis difficult. To address this issue, the American Hospital Formulary Service (AHFS) developed the Therapeutic Classification grouping system to categorize drug products. The system uses six-digit numbers that are actually three groups of two digits separated by colons, but stored in the data files as six-digit numbers without the colons. Each set of two digits provides greater specificity to the type of drug being categorized (Scerbo et al. 2001, 29). For example, Therapeutic Classification 68:00 is Hormones and synthetic substitutes, with 68:20 being Antidiabetic agents and 68:20:08 being Insulins. If the data analyst is attempting to determine whether or not diabetic patients received insulin during their stay, it would be easier to search for the Therapeutic Classification of 68:20:08 rather than all of the individual NDCs possible for every type of insulin.

Therapeutic Classification codes are available in the OVID Field Guide website (see online appendix G).

Pharmaceutical data may also be identified by RxNorm. RxNorm is a naming system for prescription and over-the-counter drugs that is produced by the National Library of Medicine (NLM). According to the NLM website, the purpose of RxNorm is to allow providers to standardize the naming conventions and identifiers for drugs. There are five steps to the creation of RxNorm, as shown in figure 2.1.

Figure 2.1   How RxNorm is produced

1. Group source data into collections of synonyms (called concepts).

Sample source data:

- Naproxen Tab 250 MG
- Naproxen 250mg tablet (product)
- NAPROXEN@250 mg@ORAL@TABLET
- Naproxen 250 MILLIGRAM In 1 TABLET ORAL TABLET
- NAPROXEN 250MG TAB,UD [VA Product]

Sources format their drug names in many different ways. Although the drug names in this Naproxen example appear different, they all have the same meaning at a certain level of abstraction. RxNorm groups these as synonyms into one concept.

2. Create an RxNorm normalized name for each concept (if the concept is in scope and unambiguous).

About 60 percent of the drug names from source vocabularies receive RxNorm normalized names in addition to the names provided by the source vocabularies. The other 40 percent do not receive RxNorm normalized names, because they are either out of scope or their names are too ambiguous. The most common types of names that are not assigned RxNorm normalized names are medical devices, foods, and enzymes.

The Naproxen concept above is in scope for RxNorm, so it is assigned an RxNorm normalized name. The normalized name consists of the ingredient, strength, and dose form (in that order) for fully-specified generic drugs. In our example, the RxNorm normalized name is 'Naproxen 250 MG Oral Tablet'. The branded version of this drug uses the same format but includes the brand name in brackets at the end (e.g., 'Naproxen 250 MG Oral Tablet [Prosaid]').

3. Assign an RxNorm concept unique identifier (RXCUI) to each concept and an RxNorm atom unique identifier (RXAUI) to each atom.

Each concept receives an RXCUI, which is unique to that concept. An RXCUI is essentially the "name" of a concept that computers read and understand. RXCUIs are never deleted or reused; RXCUIs and the meanings of concepts persist from one RxNorm release to the next.

Concepts are collections of synonyms at a given level of abstraction. Each drug name carries additional characteristics, including its source, its code (the unique identifier assigned by its source), and its term type (described below). An atom is a drug name plus these additional characteristics. Each atom within a concept receives an atom unique identifier, an RXAUI.

NLM assigns the RXCUI '198013' to the Naproxen concept above. Each of the atoms associated with the drug names listed above receives a separate RXAUI.

4. Include relationships and attributes from the source data.

Source data include more than drug names in some cases. Data can also include relationships that link drug names to other drug names and ingredients, as well as other information, such as National Drug Codes (NDCs), marketing categories, and pill imprint information.

Using the same example as before, you'll find relationships to synonyms and ingredients, as well as NDC, manufacturer, and pill size attributes.

| Figure 2.1 | *continued* |

5. Create related RxNorm names and relationships.

In addition to the fully complete clinical drug names (ingredient, strength, and dose form), RxNorm also creates names at other levels of specificity:

- ingredient / precise ingredient / multiple ingredients
- ingredient + strength
- ingredient + dose form / ingredient + dose form group

Whenever NLM creates a fully-specified drug name, these more general names (and the concepts that contain these names) are also created if they don't already exist. RxNorm then creates relationships to link these concepts together. This set of concepts and relationships is a "graph." So for both generic and branded drugs, RxNorm "fills out the graph" by creating the related drug names (and their concepts) that don't already exist. In the case of branded drugs, NLM creates their generic counterparts when they don't already exist in the data.

Along with the RxNorm fully-specified name 'Naproxen 250 MG Oral Tablet', NLM creates:

- 'Naproxen'
- 'Naproxen 250 MG'
- 'Naproxen Oral Tablet' / 'Naproxen Oral Products' / 'Naproxen Pills'

RxNorm links these names using relationships. Here are a few examples:

- 'Naproxen 250 MG Oral Tablet' has_dose_form 'Oral Tablet'
- 'Naproxen' ingredient_of 'Naproxen 250 MG'
- 'Naproxen 250 MG Oral Tablet' isa 'Naproxen Oral Tablet'
- 'Naproxen Pills' has_ingredient 'Naproxen'

Source: National Library of Medicine, 2013.

Administrative Data

Healthcare data uses several sets of codes that are not related to disease classification or treatment methods. These data sets are administrative data, or data created or collected through the registration and billing process. This section discusses the three most common sets of these codes. The first are revenue codes, which are recorded on hospital facility claims to assign services and charges to departments. Place of service codes are used on physician and and suppliers to describe where a CPT or HCPCS service has been performed. Finally, claims processing codes, such as the Medicare Code Editor (MCE) and Outpatient Code Editor (OCE) codes, are found on remittance advices to describe claims processing errors on hospital claims.

Revenue Codes

Revenue is the total of the charges generated from providing healthcare services. A **revenue code** is the four-digit number used to categorize charges on the **Uniform Bill-04 (UB-04)** claim or in the 837I electronic file associated with the claim. Although claims data is now almost exclusively submitted electronically using the 5010 format, an example of a UB-04 paper copy presented in figure 2.1 to help the reader visualize the data available on the claim form. The revenue code represents a standardized department in a facility and is required for each charge line when billing services to Medicare. The code also tracks Medicare costs by revenue centers for the Medicare cost report and categorizes revenue by similar types of services such as radiology or lab. Each hospital provider has their own internal listing of departments used in their accounting system and general ledger. Since the standard UB-04 revenue codes are required for claim submission, they allow a standardized comparison of departmental resources used to treat patients.

A complete listing of revenue codes can be found at the Research Data Assistance Center (ResDAC) website (see online appendix G). ResDAC is a CMS contractor that provides assistance to researchers and other entities that wish to access Medicare or Medicaid data for research purposes.

Place of Service Codes

These codes are used on professional claims to specify the entity or location where the service was performed. They are also used within physician practice management systems to categorize sources of revenue such as office-based services, hospital services, and nursing home services, as they form natural service classifications by site of service. A complete listing of Place of Service codes is available on their website (see online appendix G).

Claims Processing Codes

When claims are not paid or are not paid entirely, the payer reports the reasons for the lack of payment or the claim error on an Explanation of Benefits statement or a Remittance Advice using a variety of codes. These code types include:

- Claim Adjustment Reason codes: Used to communicate an adjustment or why a claim or service line was paid differently than it was billed. If there is no adjustment to a claim or line, then there is no adjustment reason code.
- Remittance Advice Remark codes: Used to convey information about remittance processing or to provide a supplemental explanation for an adjustment already described by a Claim Adjustment Reason code. Each Remittance Advice Remark code identifies a specific message as shown in the remittance advice remark code list.
- Claim status codes: Used in the Health Care Claim Status Notification (277) transaction in the STC01-2, STC10-2, and STC11-2 composite elements.

Complete listings of each code type above and the individual codes can be found on the Washington Publishing Company's website (see online appendix G).

In addition to these claims processing codes, Medicare also uses edit codes to report the reasons why hospital outpatient claims are not paid when processing through the OCE software. The complete listing of these codes and their descriptions can be found on the CMS website (see online appendix G).

Codes from these various categories are captured during the payment posting process and can provide valuable information about patterns of errors in the claims submission process. Data analysts may be asked to work with these codes to identify patterns.

Relative Value Unit Data

Relative value units (RVU) are assigned to CPT and HCPCS codes to determine the Medicare fee schedule payment. They are also used as a measure of the resource intensity required to deliver a service or procedure to a patient. RVU data for each individual CPT and HCPCS code can be found on the CMS website (see online appendix G). Scroll through the files to find the most current file, as files are revised and posted quarterly by CMS, with file extensions A through D representing the four quarters of the year. For example, RVU12A is the file for the first quarter of 2012.

This file contains far more than the title implies. In addition to the RVU data, the file provides the following for each code:

- A short description of the code
- The Part B payment status code
- The days included in the global surgical package for the code
- Information on which modifiers may be appropriate with the code

Table 2.1 reviews the coding systems used to describe the provision of healthcare in the United States, the files in which the codes can be found, and whether the codes are assigned or computed.

Table 2.1 Coding systems

Information	Coding systems	Sample format(s)	File type	Assigned or computed?
Diagnoses	International Classification of Diseases, ninth revision, Clinical Modification (ICD-9-CM)	098.10 V25.03 E932.1	UB-04 CMS-1500	Assigned
	International Classification of Diseases, tenth revision, Clinical Modification (ICD-10-CM)	M65.221 S48.011a T51.0×1	UB-04 CMS-1500 (to be implemented 10-1-2013)	Assigned
	Major diagnostic categories (MDCs)	18		Computed
	Diagnosis-related groups (CMS-DRGs)	468		Computed

(continued)

Table 2.1 Coding systems (*continued*)

Information	Coding systems	Sample format(s)	File type	Assigned or computed?
	Medicare severity-adjusted diagnosis-related groups (MS-DRGs)	981		Computed
Procedures	ICD-9-CM procedures	54.51	UB-04	Assigned
	ICD-10 Procedure Coding System (ICD-10-PCS)	ODBJ4ZZ	UB-04 (to be implemented 10-1-2013)	Assigned
	MS-DRGs	226		Computed
	Current Procedural Terminology (CPT) codes	44626 0137T	UB-04 CMS-1500	Assigned
	Healthcare Common Procedure Coding System (HCPCS) codes	A4570	UB-04 CMS-1500	Assigned
	Ambulatory payment classification (APC) group codes	0614		Computed
Drugs	National Drug Codes	00054372763	Pharmacy	Assigned
	Therapeutic Classification codes	68:20:08		Computed
Hospital administrative data	Revenue codes	0255	UB-04	Assigned
	Discharge disposition (patient status) codes	03	UB-04	Assigned
	Present on admission (POA) indicators	Y	UB-04	Assigned
Part B provider (physician) administrative data	Place of Service codes	11	CMS-1500	Assigned

Data Flow within Typical Healthcare Organizations

Hospital Inpatient Data Flow

The data flow for a hospital inpatient can begin in several different ways. Data collection starts in the registration department if patients are a direct admission from their physician's office or hospital outpatient department. Data collection begins in the emergency room if the patients arrive at the hospital, are assessed in the emergency room, and are admitted as an inpatient.

No matter where the data collection begins, the same patient demographic information is collected. This includes name, date of birth, and other identifying information necessary to identify a patient's account. If patients have been seen at the hospital prior to this visit, the information will be updated. Patients also have insurance information attached to their file. This insurance information tracks the valid insurance data associated with each hospital visit, such as the primary carrier, group number, subscriber identification, and the patient's relationship to the subscriber of the insurance. The same information is held for any secondary or tertiary insurance available for that date of service.

During the course of the inpatient stay, patient care is delivered and data is captured either in a paper record or through an electronic record system. As care is delivered and procedures are performed, charges are entered either by the nursing staff or the personnel performing the procedure. After the patient is discharged, the diagnoses associated with the care provided are coded and entered using the ICD-9-CM diagnostic system, including the associated present on admission indicator. The procedures or services performed are coded and entered using the ICD-9-CM procedure system. A DRG is then calculated, and the coded data along with additional information create a claim form. The additional information is determined by patient stay data such as the name(s) of the provider(s), location of the services performed, and dates of service. The charges for any services provided, such as laboratory or radiology tests or operating room procedures, are added to the claim form based on the fee schedule that is set up for the hospital.

Once the UB-04 claim information is properly formatted, the claim goes through a scrubber system that identifies any potential reasons for denial of a claim (comparing demographics, procedures and diagnoses, and considering any carrier-specific guidelines), flags the cases for review or correction, and suggests edits. Once these edits are corrected, the claim is sent electronically to the primary insurance carrier. This carrier pays the claim according to the carrier's claims payment rules and sends a **remittance advice** to the hospital detailing how the claim was paid, along with a check or electronic funds transfer for the appropriate payment. For Medicare, the Medicare Code Editor tests the claim for possible problems. If any charges are paid differently than expected, an edit message or denial code is found in the payment detail. If there is an open balance on the claim and the patient has secondary or tertiary insurance, the claim is sent to the secondary insurer and then to the tertiary insurer until all benefits due have been paid. At that time, the patient is sent a statement detailing the final balance. If the patient pays the final balance, the claim is closed (fully paid).

If the patient does not pay the balance, collection attempts are made until all efforts are exhausted. At that time, the balance is written off as bad debt.

Data is collected in the claims history at each point in the process. ICD-9-CM codes are entered as line items along with a posting date, similar to the way the codes appear on a claim form. Each action that takes place is logged in the claims file, such as payment from primary, secondary, or tertiary insurance; edit or denial codes that accompany the payment; and the amount paid by the patient. Most data systems allow retrieval of each of these data elements in the form of a report for claims follow-up or data analysis.

Hospital Outpatient Data Flow

The data flow for a hospital outpatient can begin in several different places. Patients usually have an order from their physician to have a test or procedure performed. In most cases, the data collection begins over the phone with a pre registration phone call. At this time, the patient demographic file is created with the patient's name, address, date of birth, and other identifying information necessary to identify the patient's account. An appointment is then usually made. Other data collection begins in the registration department when patients walk in with an order from their physician. Their demographic data is collected, and they proceed to the department where their test or procedure is being performed. Some data collection begins in the emergency room, where a patient demographic file is created. Along with the demographic data, insurance information is collected, including the primary carrier, group number, subscriber information, and the patient's relationship to the subscriber of the insurance. The same information is held for any secondary or tertiary insurance available for that date of service.

Patient care is delivered and data is captured either on paper or through electronic systems. In either case, the diagnoses associated with the care provided are coded and entered using the ICD-9-CM diagnostic system. The services provided are coded and entered using the CPT or HCPCS coding systems. Additional information is then added to this coded data to form a claim form. The additional information is determined by appointment data such as the name of the provider, location of care, and date of service.

The charges for the service are added to the file based on the Charge Description Master (CDM). The CDM is a complete listing of the services that may be provided to a patient and the charge for that service. The CDM itemcode is a unique identifier for the service billed. The number of units of each service is recorded for each patient and later included on the patient claim submitted for payment. For example, if two units of blood were provided, the charge in the fee schedule is multiplied by two and listed on the claim.

Additional information may be required at the time of service such as whether the service was related to an occupational injury or automobile accident. Any services provided on that day, such as radiology or laboratory tests, as well as ICD-9-CM and CPT and HCPCS codes and the number of the tests (units) performed, are also added to the claim.

Once the UB-04 claim form or the electronically submitted 837 format record has been properly formatted, the claim goes through a scrubber system to identify any edits or potential denial codes. Once the edits are corrected or the charge is submitted for write-off or removal from the claim by the hospital, the claim is sent electronically to the primary insurance carrier. This carrier pays the claim according to the carrier's claims payment rules and sends a remittance advice to the hospital detailing how each code was paid, along with a check or electronic funds transfer for the appropriate payment. If any charges are paid differently than expected, an edit message or denial code is found in the payment detail. If there is an open balance on the claim and the patient has secondary or tertiary insurance, the claim is sent to the secondary insurer and then to the tertiary insurer until all benefits due have been paid. At that time, the patient is sent a statement detailing the final balance. If the patient pays the final balance, the claim is closed (fully paid). If the patient does not pay the balance, collection attempts are made until all efforts are exhausted. At that time, the balance is written off as bad debt.

Data is collected in the claims history at each point in this process. ICD-9-CM and CPT and HCPCS codes are entered as line items along with a posting date, similar to the codes that appear on a claim form. Each action that takes place is logged in the claims database, such as payment from primary, secondary, or tertiary insurance; edit or denial codes that accompany the payment; and the amount paid by the patient. Most data systems allow retrieval of each of these data elements in the form of reports for claims follow-up or data analysis.

Physician Practice Data Flow

The data flow in a physician office is more straightforward than in any other healthcare setting. Data collection begins with the creation of an appointment date and time with a specific provider. In most practice management systems, this forms the basic shell around which all data are captured for this event.

All patients have a demographic file containing their name, address, date of birth, and other information necessary to identify their account. This file is normally updated at each appointment. A partner file on insurance information tracks the valid insurance data associated with each appointment, such as the primary carrier, group number, subscriber identification, and the patient's relationship to the subscriber of the insurance. The same information is held for any secondary or tertiary insurance available for that date of service.

Patient care is delivered and data is captured either on paper or through electronic systems. In either case, the diagnoses associated with the care provided are coded and entered using the ICD-9-CM diagnostic system. The services provided are coded and entered using the CPT and HCPCS coding systems. As the diagnosis and procedure information are entered, each service is linked to the diagnosis that supports the medical necessity for the service. Additional information is then added to this coded data to form a claim form. The additional information is determined by the appointment information, such as the name of the provider, location of care, and date of service.

The charges for the service are added to the file based on the amount that is set up for the CPT or HCPCS code, any modifiers that may have been assigned, and the number of services that were performed. For example, if three units of medication were provided, the charge in the fee schedule is multiplied by three and listed on the claim.

Additional information may be required at the time the service was entered into the computer, such as whether the service was related to an occupational injury or automobile accident, so that the primary payer can be correctly determined for these services. If other services are provided that day, such as laboratory or radiology tests, ICD-9-CM and CPT and HCPCS codes and the units of the test performed are added to the claim as well.

Once the CMS-1500 claim form is properly formatted, the claim is sent, either electronically or on paper, to the primary insurance carrier. This carrier pays the claim according to the carrier's claims payment rules and sends a remittance advice to the physician detailing how each code was paid, along with a check or electronic funds transfer for the appropriate payment. If any charges are paid differently than expected, an edit message or denial code is found in the payment detail. If there is an open balance on the claim and the patient has secondary or tertiary insurance, the claim is sent in order to these insurers until all benefits due have been paid. At that time, the patient is sent a statement detailing the final balance. If the patient pays the final balance, the claim is closed as fully paid. If the patient does not pay the balance, collection attempts are made until all efforts are exhausted. At that time, the balance is written off as bad debt.

Data is collected in the claims history at each point in this process. ICD-9-CM and CPT and HCPCS codes are entered as line items along with a posting date, similar to the codes that appear on a claim form. Each action that takes place is logged in the claims file, such as payment from primary, secondary, or tertiary insurance; edit or denial codes that accompany the payment; and the amount paid by the patient. Most data systems allow retrieval of each of these data elements in the form of reports for claims follow-up or data analysis.

Sources of Data

Data are available from sources within the organization or from sources outside the organization. Data available from inside a healthcare organization is known as internal data and can take the form of coded data in departmental systems, as well as billing data in the UB-04 and CMS-1500 files. Many facilities also have registry or discrete data from an electronic health record available for use in the data analysis process.

Internal Data

As discussed above, healthcare organizations maintain many databases that contain many different types of data. Data analysts are frequently asked to compare this data with data from other sources for benchmarking (discussed in chapter 9) or other quality improvement efforts.

Many healthcare organizations are comprised of multiple facilities, and comparative data from another facility in the same health system is readily available to all facilities within the system. Using this data, data analysts can compare facilities to each other and to the combined totals of the entire healthcare system.

Many physician groups also have the ability to share data within a larger organization. As a result, comparisons can be drawn between the physician and all of the physician's colleagues at the same location or between the physician and the physician's colleagues within the same specialty. In addition, one physician can be compared to the combined totals of the entire physician group.

Hospitals also have the opportunity to compare data from various source systems. For example, the health information management (HIM) department may have data related to outpatient surgery encounters, and a physician practice division may have professional fee data about those same outpatient surgery encounters in a practice management system. Hospitals and large clinics also may have access to data that is stored in departmental systems such as a laboratory information system (LIS) or in the cardiology lab or endoscopy lab. In addition, the HIM system and other departmental systems feed charges to the facility billing system, whose data may not be found in any other system. The department data may be fed into an enterprise-wide database that combines data for all departments so that the complete profile of a patient encounter may be presented in one location. The level of data integration at a provider site will impact the amount of data acquisition and combining that might be required of an analyst prior to preforming the actual statistical analysis of the data.

Systems within healthcare organizations are frequently interfaced, and data analysts are often called upon to determine why data from one system is not exactly the same as data housed in another system. The data analyst can play an important role in determining if data interfaces are functioning properly and can suggest where interface issues may be located. The topics of validating the integrity of data interfaces and the data in various departmental systems will be discussed further in chapter 9.

Claims Data

A healthcare claim is an itemized statement of healthcare services and their costs provided by the hospital, physician office, or other healthcare provider. Claims are submitted for reimbursement to the insurance plan by the provider using two different formats, depending upon the type of service that was provided.

UB-04 (CMS-1450) Claim Form

Institutional or facility-based services are submitted using the UB-04 data set. A fact sheet on the completion of this data set can be found and instructions for completing and processing the UB-04 (CMS-1450) data set is available on the CMS website (see online appendix G).

Data in the UB-04 data set is grouped by field locator numbers that indicate the placement of the data on the form and in the associated electronic transaction file. Figure 2.1 displays the printed version of the UB-04, also called the CMS-1450 form.

The information contained on the UB-04 is transmitted to many healthcare payers using the 837I transaction set via the 5010 format. The format and details on this electronic record may be found on the CMS website (see online appendix G).

CMS-1500 Claim Form

Professional fee claims are submitted using the CMS-1500 data set that describes services by physicians and other healthcare professionals. Instructions for completing and processing the CMS-1500 data set are available on the CMS website (see online appendix G).

Data in the CMS-1500 data set are organized by block numbers or item numbers. Table 2.2 shows the block names associated with the CMS-1500 data set, and figure 2.2 displays the printed version of the CMS-1500 form. The electronically submitted version of the CMS-1500 is transmitted using the 837P standard format. The details on that format may be found on the CMS website (see online appendix G).

Figure 2.2 **UB-04 (CMS-1450) claim form**

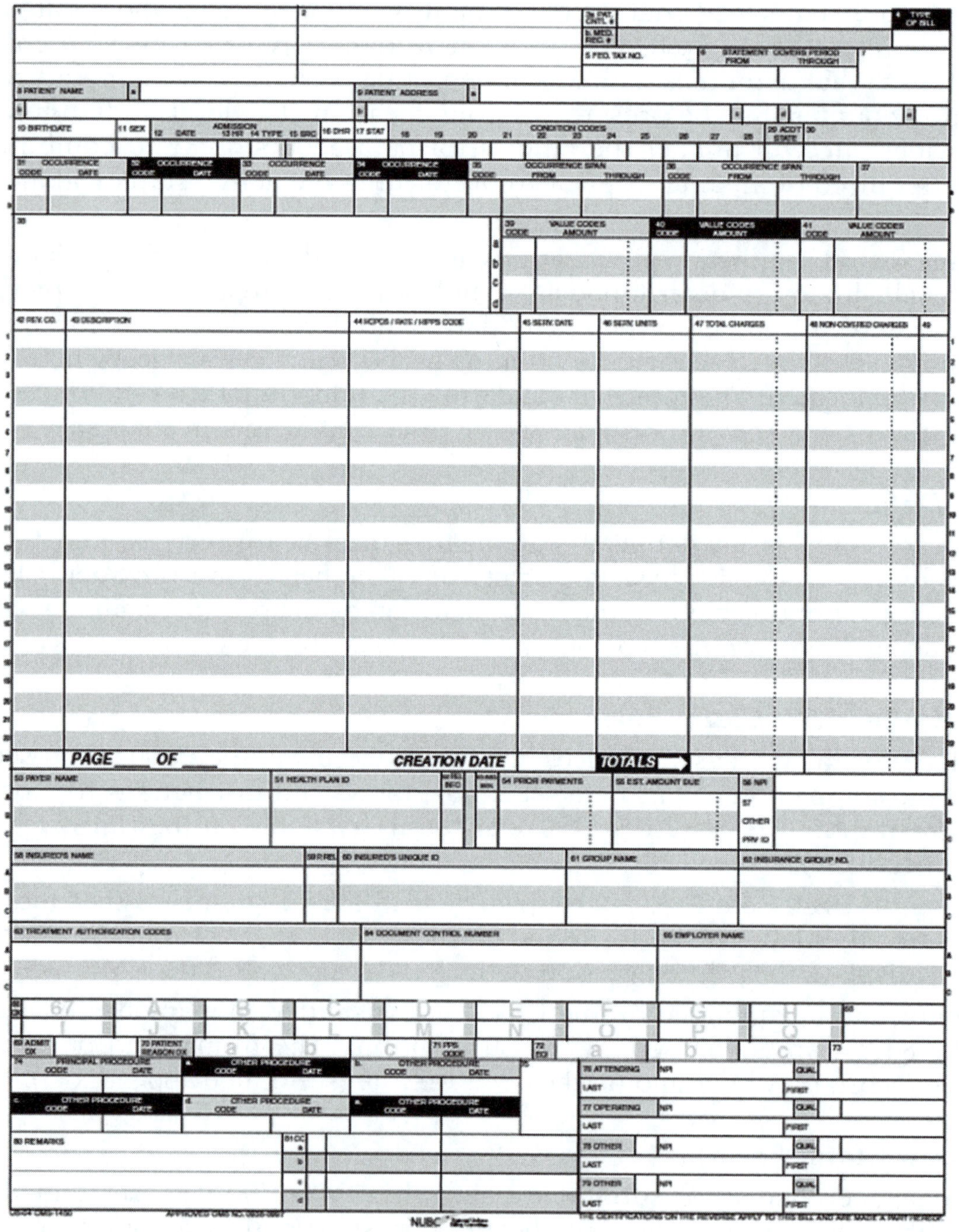

Table 2.2 CMS-1500 blocks

Block #	Brief Description	Block #	Brief Description
1	Type of insurance	19	Reserved for local use
1a	Insured's ID number	20	Outside lab
2	Patient's name	21	Diagnosis pointer (Reference Number from Block 21)
3	Patient's birthdate/sex	22	Medicaid resubmission
4	Insured's name	23	Prior authorization number
5	Patient's address	24A	Dates of service
6	Patient's relationship to insured	24B	Place of service
7	Insured's address	24C	EMG
8	Patient's marital status/employment status	24D	Procedures, services, or supplies
9	Other insured's name	24E	Diagnosis code
9a	Other insured's policy or group number	24F	Charges
9b	Other insured's date of birth/sex	24G	Days or units
9c	Employer's name or school name	24H	EPSDT family plan
9d	Insurance plan name or program name	24I	ID qualifier
10a–10c	Indicate whether patient's condition is related to a work injury, an automobile accident, or another type of accident	24J	Rendering provider ID #
10d	Reserved for local use		
11	Insured's policy group or FECA number	25	Federal tax ID number
11a	Insured's date of birth/sex	26	Patient's account number
11b	Employer's name or school name	27	Accept assignment or not
11c	Insurance plan name or program name of insured	28	Total charge
11d	Indicate whether there is another health benefit plan	29	Amount paid
12	Patient's or authorized person's signature	30	Balance due
13	Insured or authorized person's signature	31	Signature of physician or supplier

(continued)

Table 2.2 CMS-1500 blocks (*continued*)

Block #	Brief Description	Block #	Brief Description
14	Date of current illness or injury or pregnancy	32	Service facility location information
15	Date when patient first consulted provider for treatment of the same or similar condition	32a	NPI
16	Dates patient unable to work in current occupation	32b	Provider PIN for certain services
17	Name of referring physician or other source	33	Billing provider info and phone number
17a	ID number of referring physician	33a	NPI
17b	NPI	33b	National supplier clearinghouse number for DMERC or provider PIN
18	Hospitalization dates related to current services		

Departmental Databases

Healthcare organizations collect and use data at all points in the delivery of healthcare. This data collection and manipulation has highly specialized requirements and, therefore, specialized databases or software systems are maintained for this purpose. This section discusses the most common databases found in healthcare organizations. Facilities may have an enterprise-wide data system that combines the data traditionally found in these departmental databases. The content of the departmental packages of the enterprise-wide database or EHR system is similar to that listed in the following sections. The querying and combining of the data is much easier when an enterprise-wide database exists.

Health Information Management Database

This specialized database contains the coded data assigned to the diagnoses and procedures associated with each hospital inpatient service. Some hospitals also capture data on outpatient services using this system, but this is not universal. The database works with software, known as a grouper, that assigns hospital discharges to an MDC and an MS-DRG within that MDC. A grouper for assigning APCs to outpatient services may also be associated with this database.

Common features of this database are the ability to determine that all records have been coded and submitted to the patient accounts database and edits that alert HIM staff of data entry errors or incongruities.

Data analysts would query this database for details of the stay that are not used to generate a claim, such as the name of a surgeon who performed a specific procedure at a specific operative setting during the inpatient stay.

Figure 2.3 CMS-1500 claim form

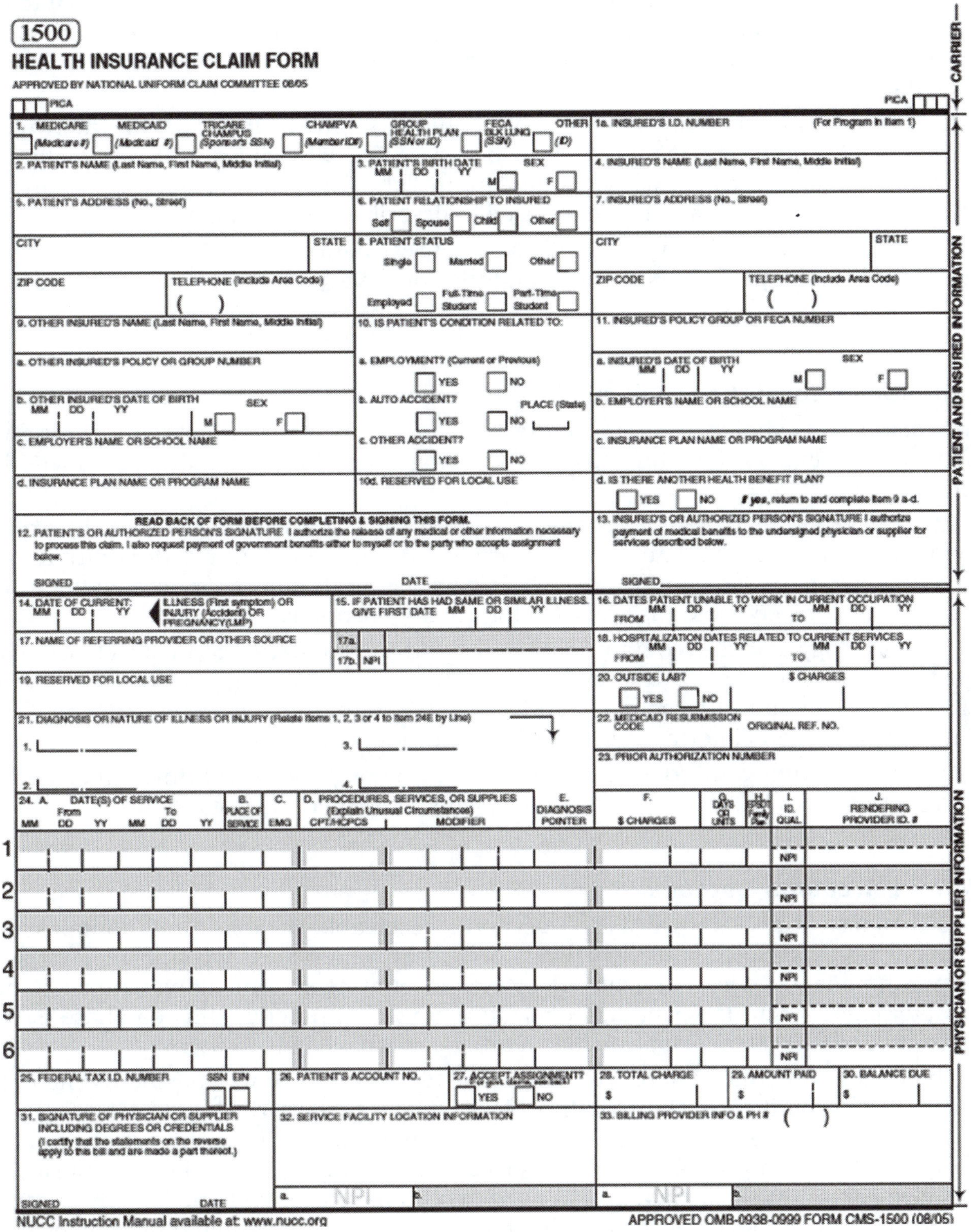

1500

HEALTH INSURANCE CLAIM FORM

APPROVED BY NATIONAL UNIFORM CLAIM COMMITTEE 08/05

PICA PICA

CARRIER

1. MEDICARE (Medicare #) MEDICAID (Medicaid #) TRICARE CHAMPUS (Sponsor's SSN) CHAMPVA (Member ID#) GROUP HEALTH PLAN (SSN or ID) FECA BLK LUNG (SSN) OTHER (ID)

1a. INSURED'S I.D. NUMBER (For Program in Item 1)

2. PATIENT'S NAME (Last Name, First Name, Middle Initial)

3. PATIENT'S BIRTH DATE MM DD YY SEX M F

4. INSURED'S NAME (Last Name, First Name, Middle Initial)

5. PATIENT'S ADDRESS (No., Street)

6. PATIENT RELATIONSHIP TO INSURED Self Spouse Child Other

7. INSURED'S ADDRESS (No., Street)

CITY STATE

8. PATIENT STATUS Single Married Other

CITY STATE

ZIP CODE TELEPHONE (Include Area Code) ( )

Employed Full-Time Student Part-Time Student

ZIP CODE TELEPHONE (Include Area Code) ( )

9. OTHER INSURED'S NAME (Last Name, First Name, Middle Initial)

10. IS PATIENT'S CONDITION RELATED TO:

11. INSURED'S POLICY GROUP OR FECA NUMBER

a. OTHER INSURED'S POLICY OR GROUP NUMBER

a. EMPLOYMENT? (Current or Previous) YES NO

a. INSURED'S DATE OF BIRTH MM DD YY SEX M F

b. OTHER INSURED'S DATE OF BIRTH MM DD YY SEX M F

b. AUTO ACCIDENT? YES NO PLACE (State)

b. EMPLOYER'S NAME OR SCHOOL NAME

c. EMPLOYER'S NAME OR SCHOOL NAME

c. OTHER ACCIDENT? YES NO

c. INSURANCE PLAN NAME OR PROGRAM NAME

d. INSURANCE PLAN NAME OR PROGRAM NAME

10d. RESERVED FOR LOCAL USE

d. IS THERE ANOTHER HEALTH BENEFIT PLAN? YES NO *If yes*, return to and complete item 9 a-d.

READ BACK OF FORM BEFORE COMPLETING & SIGNING THIS FORM.

12. PATIENT'S OR AUTHORIZED PERSON'S SIGNATURE I authorize the release of any medical or other information necessary to process this claim. I also request payment of government benefits either to myself or to the party who accepts assignment below.

SIGNED DATE

13. INSURED'S OR AUTHORIZED PERSON'S SIGNATURE I authorize payment of medical benefits to the undersigned physician or supplier for services described below.

SIGNED

PATIENT AND INSURED INFORMATION

14. DATE OF CURRENT: MM DD YY ILLNESS (First symptom) OR INJURY (Accident) OR PREGNANCY(LMP)

15. IF PATIENT HAS HAD SAME OR SIMILAR ILLNESS. GIVE FIRST DATE MM DD YY

16. DATES PATIENT UNABLE TO WORK IN CURRENT OCCUPATION FROM MM DD YY TO MM DD YY

17. NAME OF REFERRING PROVIDER OR OTHER SOURCE 17a. 17b. NPI

18. HOSPITALIZATION DATES RELATED TO CURRENT SERVICES FROM MM DD YY TO MM DD YY

19. RESERVED FOR LOCAL USE

20. OUTSIDE LAB? YES NO $ CHARGES

21. DIAGNOSIS OR NATURE OF ILLNESS OR INJURY (Relate Items 1, 2, 3 or 4 to Item 24E by Line)

1. 2. 3. 4.

22. MEDICAID RESUBMISSION CODE ORIGINAL REF. NO.

23. PRIOR AUTHORIZATION NUMBER

24. A. DATE(S) OF SERVICE From MM DD YY To MM DD YY	B. PLACE OF SERVICE	C. EMG	D. PROCEDURES, SERVICES, OR SUPPLIES (Explain Unusual Circumstances) CPT/HCPCS MODIFIER	E. DIAGNOSIS POINTER	F. $ CHARGES	G. DAYS OR UNITS	H. EPSDT Family Plan	I. ID. QUAL.	J. RENDERING PROVIDER ID. #
1								NPI	
2								NPI	
3								NPI	
4								NPI	
5								NPI	
6								NPI	

25. FEDERAL TAX I.D. NUMBER SSN EIN

26. PATIENT'S ACCOUNT NO.

27. ACCEPT ASSIGNMENT? (For govt. claims, see back) YES NO

28. TOTAL CHARGE $

29. AMOUNT PAID $

30. BALANCE DUE $

31. SIGNATURE OF PHYSICIAN OR SUPPLIER INCLUDING DEGREES OR CREDENTIALS (I certify that the statements on the reverse apply to this bill and are made a part thereof.)

SIGNED DATE

32. SERVICE FACILITY LOCATION INFORMATION

a. NPI b.

33. BILLING PROVIDER INFO & PH # ( )

a. NPI b.

PHYSICIAN OR SUPPLIER INFORMATION

NUCC Instruction Manual available at: www.nucc.org

APPROVED OMB-0938-0999 FORM CMS-1500 (08/05)

Laboratory Information System (LIS) Database

This database contains information on laboratory tests; including order and specimen tracking, result values, report formats, and billing data. This is a complex database that is often interfaced to actual laboratory test machines and to the patient accounts database for billing. Information on the staff that performed each operation is also typically available.

Data stored in this database normally contain **Logical Observation Identifiers Names and Codes (LOINC)**. These codes describe lab values and other clinical observations. They are the exchange standard for laboratory results and are used in the database in addition to the CPT codes used to describe the test name.

Data analysts would query this database to retrieve data on order times, result values, professionals who performed the test, and the combination of tests that were ordered and performed.

Radiology Information System (RIS) Database

This database is similar to a laboratory information system but contains additional data about patient scheduling, patient tracking, and the staff that performed the actual exam.

In radiology, the patient must be present during the examination. This makes appointment and exam-length data important information to track. In addition, not all radiology images are completed correctly on the first exam. Therefore, data on the percentage of image retakes is recorded for quality purposes.

The radiology database contains the results of the examination as unstructured data after the images are read by the radiologist. The actual image may be available in the RIS through the use of a picture archiving and communication system (PACS). This database is normally interfaced to the patient accounts database.

Data analysts query this database to retrieve data on appointment times and lengths, number of images taken, and professionals who performed the tests.

Patient Accounts Database

This database is also known as the accounts receivable database and contains the financial data associated with the delivery of healthcare services. Accounts receivable is a key component of the organization's overall accounting system, along with accounts payable, payroll, and the general ledger. In a physician practice, this database is the heart of the data system, usually called a practice management system.

The patient accounts database contains the demographic data and the billing data necessary to submit one or both of the different claim types (UB-04 and CMS-1500) for the organization. Demographic data may be entered directly into a registration table of this database, while billing data is received in other ways. The HIM data is normally sent electronically to this database after the codes have been assigned to the services that have been provided. Departmental charge data are either entered directly or sent electronically.

Codes describing the outcome of the claims submission process, known as Medicare Code Editor (MCE) codes or Outpatient Code Editor (OCE) codes, are normally found in this database on the CMS website (see appendix G). The editor codes describe any reasons why the claim was returned to the provider for correction or not paid as expected. In addition, the OCE code specifies which action should be taken and the reasons why these actions are necessary to complete the processing of the claim. Additional information on OCE codes can be found in chapter 6.

Data analysts would query this database for claims data, patient demographics, and claims processing codes.

Clinical Data Repository (CDR)

The CDR is a type of database that organizes data from many different sources and makes it readily available to users. Data that go into a repository may come from various source systems or may be entered by a user directly. Data in a CDR may be structured, or "discrete," data or it may be unstructured data. Clinical data repositories are normally built from a variety of data sources and input, including direct entry and interfaced systems, which are discussed earlier in this chapter.

Unstructured data includes narrative notes as well as images (of scanned documents or medical images). (LaTour and Eichenwald-Maki 2013, 118). This data may be entered directly by the clinician, or interfaced to the CDR from another system (such as transcription, dictation, or radiology).

Discrete data may enter the CDR from departmental systems or from clinical systems such as an electronic medication administration record (eMAR) or patient care charting system. These systems collect discrete data elements that cannot be coded using a standard classification system but are important to understanding the delivery of healthcare. The eMAR is the primary data source for exact administration time and identification of the administering staff member. The patient care charting system in a hospital or the electronic health record in a physician office are the primary data sources on patient vital signs such as height, weight, blood pressure, or temperature at a given date and time during the stay.

The type of data, structured or unstructured, found in the CDR will determine the level and types of analyses that can be performed using the data. Unstructured data may be profiled and summarized using qualitative analysis. Discrete data elements may be analyzed using traditional quantitative analysis such as descriptive and inferential statistics.

Other Data

Healthcare organizations may maintain data in other locations for specific reasons, such as in subject-based databases or registries. Some of the most common registries maintained are as follows:

- Cancer (tumor)
- Trauma
- Birth defects

- Diabetes
- Implants
- Transplants
- Immunizations

In addition to codes, these registries contain valuable information pertinent to the subject of the registry. For example, a cancer registry includes staging of the disease at the time of diagnosis, treatment protocols, the industrial or occupational history of the patient, survival status, and quality-of-life information. All of these pieces of information could be extremely helpful to a data analyst working on a related topic (LaTour and Eichenwald-Maki 2013, 370–372).

Note that both an implant registry and an immunization registry maintain information specific to the manufacturer of the registry's product to facilitate patient notification in the event of a product recall for any reason. All of these registries may also have state or regional counterparts used to collect data and share information on a larger population.

With the implementation of recovery audit contractors (RACs), facilities are beginning to develop databases that track all of the issues related to claims denials by the RACs. These databases can track reasons for the denials as well as timing and processing of the claims through the appeals process.

External Data

External data may take the form of claims data that have been submitted to a government payer or quality data that have been submitted to a regulatory body or other agency. (Quality indicator data will be discussed in chapter 9.) This section discusses data that are not facility-specific and that are available from CMS and various state governments.

Medicare

CMS provides public use data files that may be used for research and benchmarking purposes. A brief description of the files is included in the following section. More details regarding Medicare data that is available and the process for obtaining the data may be found on the CMS website (see online appendix G).

Medicare Provider Analysis and Review (MedPAR)

The Medicare Provider Analysis and Review (MedPAR) file contains data from claims for services provided to beneficiaries admitted to Medicare-certified inpatient hospitals and skilled nursing facilities. MEDPAR files contain information for 100 percent of Medicare beneficiaries using hospital inpatient services. A summary of the annual MedPAR file is provided by state and then by DRG for all short-stay and inpatient hospitals and is available for download from the CMS website (see online appendix G). The file contains the following information by DRG: total charges, covered charges, Medicare reimbursement, total days (length of stay), number of discharges, and average total days.

Hospital Outpatient Data

CMS has outpatient data in its standard outpatient analytical file (SAOF) that can be requested based on multiple parameters. This is identifiable data, and privacy approval must be given first. In addition, there is a fee associated with the provision of this data, and it is not available for immediate download. It is available only on request and approval of a defined research plan for the data by CMS.

Also note that each year's Hospital Outpatient Prospective Payment System files include the Medicare hospital outpatient claims that are used to set the APC payments each year. This is a limited data set and requires a data use agreement to be signed with CMS as well as a defined research plan prior to obtaining the file. These files are available on the CMS website and are organized by year (see online appendix G). Volume of services by CPT code and the estimated cost of services may be found in the OPPS rule released annually by CMS.

Part B Utilization Data

The CMS website contains links to Medicare Part B utilization data that can be useful for comparison. This data can be found in the Research, Statistics, Data and Systems section of the site under "Medicare Fee for Service for Parts A & B." Choose "Medicare Utilization for Part B" when using the menu system on the CMS website (see online appendix G).

The files contain data on the most frequently used codes, Evaluation and Management (E/M) code frequencies by specialty and expenditures, and services by specialty. Some topics are organized by the amount of charges submitted, and some are organized by the number of services submitted. Data from 2011 is the most recent data available at the time of publication.

State Databases

Many states have volumes of data on their websites. Most states provide standard reports that include data in commonly requested combinations. Utah and Massachusetts are two states that have data that can be queried by the user.

Utah

The Utah Health Data Committee of the Office of Health Care Statistics provides a variety of different data reports regarding healthcare in Utah. Reports are available on hospital utilization, hospital and ambulatory surgery center utilization, and pharmacy utilization. These formatted reports are available on their website (see online appendix G).

In addition, Utah provides three query tools for use in locating specific data from the Utah databases. These query tools search on descriptive statistics, hospitalization rates, and external cases of injury and are found on their website (see appendix G). No downloading of software is required.

Massachusetts

The Massachusetts Community Health Information Profile, or MassCHIP, has standard reports called Instant Topics, available on their website (see online appendix G).

MassCHIP also has downloadable query software to allow users to query the database for custom reports.

Other Organizations

Other private and government-sponsored programs collect data and report it back to users in an organized fashion. Some of this data are publicly available, and some are available for purchase.

The Healthcare Cost and Utilization Project (HCUP)

The Healthcare Cost and Utilization Project (HCUP) sponsors HCUPnet on the web. HCUPnet is an online query system that provides instant access to the largest set of all-payer healthcare databases that are publicly available. Using HCUPnet's query system, you can generate tables and graphs on national and regional statistics and trends for community hospitals in the United States. In addition, community hospital data are available for those states that have agreed to participate in HCUPnet. HCUP supports the following data sets:

- National Inpatient Sample (NIS) – all payer inpatient data
- Kids' Inpatient Database (KID) – pediatric inpatient data
- Nationwide Emergency Department Sample (NEDS) – all payer emergency department data
- State Inpatient Databases (SID) – all payer data for selected states
- State Ambulatory Surgery Databases (SASD) – all payer data for selected states
- State Emergency Department Databases (SEDD) – all payer data for selected states

The NIS, KID, and NEDS are all databases that support all patient projections based on a sample from the statewide databases and selected providers. The SID, SASD, and SEDD are all based on all payer databases that are collected in a number of states. They include all of the records submitted and are not projections based on a sample.

These files are available for query on the HCUPnet website (see online appendix G). The majority of the files are free, but files that can be queried for highly specific data must be purchased for a fee. Using the menu system can be complicated, but the tool is powerful. To see how the system works, consider an example exercise that involves retrieving data about ICD-9-CM 38.44, resection with replacement of the abdominal aorta, an ICD-9-CM procedure code in 2010. Remember to select codes that are valid during the year in which data is being requested.

To retrieve the report from our example exercise, click on the following options:

- National Statistics on All Stays
- Researcher, medical professional
- Statistics on specific diagnoses or procedures
- 2010 Specific procedures by ICD-9-CM
- Principal procedure
- 3844 (enter 3844 in the box)

Figure 2.4 HCUP data on resection with replacement of the abdominal aorta

2010 National statistics - principal procedure only

Outcomes by patient and hospital characteristics for ICD-9-CM principal procedure code 38.44
Resect Abdm Aorta W Repl

		Total number of discharges	LOS (length of stay), days (mean)	Standard errors	
				Total number of discharges	LOS (length of stay), days (mean)
All discharges		9,561 (100.00%)	11.3	785	0.4
Region	Northeast	1,852 (19.37%)	11.8	381	1.1
	Midwest	2,660 (27.82%)	11.4	497	0.6
	South	3,508 (36.69%)	11.3	421	0.7
	West	1,540 (16.11%)	10.6	215	0.7

Weighted national estimates from HCUP Nationwide Inpatient Sample (NIS), 2010, Agency for Healthcare Research and Quality (AHRQ), based on data collected by individual States and provided to AHRQ by the States. Total number of weighted discharges in the U.S. based on HCUP NIS = 39,008,298. Statistics based on estimates with a relative standard error (standard error / weighted estimate) greater than 0.30 or with standard error = 0 in the nationwide statistics (NIS,NEDS, and KID) are not reliable. These statistics are suppressed and are designated with an asterisk (*). The estimates of standard errors in HCUPnet were calculated using SUDAAN software. These estimates may differ slightly if other software packages are used to calculate variances.

If you want to test whether apparent differences are significant, use the Z-Test Calculator. A p -value of less than 0.05 is generally considered statistically significant.

Source: *The Healthcare Cost and Utilization Project (HCUP)*

- Number of Discharges and Length of Stay, Mean
- Region of the United States

Then the report will be displayed. Click "save as an Excel spreadsheet" if you want to save the data for future use or manipulation.

Figure 2.4 is the report that results when the parameters described on the previous page are chosen.

Medical Group Management Association (MGMA)

The Medical Group Management Association (MGMA) is a professional association for executives within physician practices. MGMA has recognized that finding national comparative data for physicians from a source other than CMS is extremely difficult. To address this issue, the association developed a confidential data collection service and has published national comparative data since 2003, entitled *Coding Profile Sourcebooks*. This data is available for purchase on an interactive CD. It provides information on all common specialties as well as additional software for data analysis that allows the export of extracted data into Excel spreadsheets. Data is available for patients of all ages and for specialties that are normally not represented or categorized well in CMS data, such as pediatrics and hospitalists. Data is available at a considerably lower price to members of the association and is found on the MGMA website (see online appendix G).

 Review Questions

1. DRGs may be grouped into:
   a. Major Diagnostic Categories
   b. Procedural categories
   c. Clinical modifications
   d. CMS-DRGs

2. MS-DRG is an acronym for:
   a. Medical standard diagnosis related groups
   b. Medicare severity diagnosis related groups
   c. Medical society diagnosis related groups
   d. Medicare standardized diagnosis related groups

3. Which of the following is not a type of procedure code?
   a. ICD-10-PCS
   b. CPT
   c. DRG
   d. HCPCS

4. A revenue code represents a:
   a. Facility department
   b. Reason for a claim denial
   c. Amount charged for a service
   d. Diagnostic code

5. Relative value units are used to:
   a. Determine payment for physician services
   b. Describe procedures performed in a hospital
   c. Report a claim status
   d. Report the reason for the denial of payment for a service

6. Which of the following represents data flow for a hospital inpatient admission?
   a. Registration > diagnostic and procedure codes assigned > services performed > charges recorded
   b. Registration > services performed > charges recorded > diagnostic and procedure codes assigned

    c. Services performed > charges recorded > registration > diagnostic and procedure codes assigned

    d. Diagnostic and procedure codes assigned > registration > services performed > charges recorded

7. Which of the following is the correct claim form for inpatient hospital claims?

    a. CMS-1450

    b. Remittance advice

    c. MS-DRG

    d. CMS-1500

8. Which of the following is the correct claim form for physician claims?

    a. CMS-1450

    b. Remittance advice

    c. MS-DRG

    d. CMS-1500

9. LOINC is primarily a coding system for:

    a. Drugs

    b. Diagnoses

    c. Physician specialty

    d. Laboratory values

10. The MedPAR file contains what type of data?

    a. Physician claims

    b. Outpatient claims

    c. Inpatient claims

    d. Hospital census data

📖 References

Kuehn, L. 2013. *Procedural Coding and Reimbursement for Physician Services: Applying Current Procedural Terminology and HCPCS*. Chicago: AHIMA.

LaTour, K.M. and S. Eichenwald-Maki. 2013. *Health Information Management Concepts, Principles and Practice*, 4th ed. Chicago: AHIMA.

National Library of Medicine. 2013. RxNorm Overview. http://www.nlm.nih.gov/research/umls/rxnorm/overview.html

Scerbo, M., C. Dickstein, and A. Wilson. 2001. *Health Care Data and SAS*. Cary, NC: SAS Institute Inc.

Tools for Data Organization, Analysis, and Presentation

KEY TERMS

Data dictionary
Database
Entity relationship diagram
Healthcare Effectiveness Data and
Information Set (HEDIS)
Query

Relational database management
system
Structured query language (SQL)
Statistical Analysis System (SAS)
Statistical Package for the Social
Sciences (SPSS)

Data Organization Using Databases

A **database** is a self-describing collection of integrated records. Each record has multiple attributes, and each attribute has one or more values per entry. The database is self-describing because it contains a description of its own structure, and it is integrated because it has a relationship between the data items.

Relational databases are a two-dimensional array of rows and columns, containing single-valued entries with no duplicate rows. Each cell in the array can have only one value, and no two rows can be identical (Taylor 2006, 8).

This chapter presents a general overview of data tools. A more in-depth presentation of database concepts may be found in appendix A.

Small-Scale Databases

Microsoft Office Access is a **relational database management system** from Microsoft that is very versatile for development. Skilled software developers and data architects can use it to develop robust applications, while relatively unskilled programmers can use it to build simple applications or customized databases for limited use or manipulation of data. Access is part of the Microsoft Office package and is therefore commonly available to many PC users. Access database files have an extension of .mdb for Access 2003 or .accdb for Access 2007/2010/2013.

Access is best used by a single user or only a few users because it includes limited functionality for user support and control. Once multiple users need to work with the data simultaneously, database designers typically prefer to build databases and applications in Microsoft structured query language (SQL) Server, Oracle, or other database products. However, for small databases, Access does have the advantages of a relatively quick development time and a graphic user interface that uses a query design grid to create queries that are compatible with SQL (pronounced "ess-que-ell" or "sequel"). Due to these advantages, data that is stored in other database programs can be imported or linked into Microsoft Access for easier manipulation.

Complex Data in Large or Multiple Databases

When databases are large or part of a scheme of multiple databases, an **entity relationship diagram (ERD)** is used to describe how the tables work together. The diagram is a graphic representation of the entities, attributes, and relationships that are part of a database and is a data modeling tool.

An entity is something about which data are collected. The entity is synonymous for the table names found in a database.

Attributes are the characteristics or data elements to be collected about each entity or table. The titles of the attributes are usually maintained in the form of lists. An attribute whose value is based on the value of other attributes in known as a derived variable. The classic example is the derived attribute of age, calculated as the current date field minus the date-of-birth field.

An attribute that is a unique identifier in a table is called the primary key. The primary key cannot be duplicated within the table and cannot contain a null value (be empty). Keys are repeated in different tables to link tables together. When a primary key is duplicated in another table, it is called a foreign key.

Figure 3.1 shows the hierarchy of a relational database.

Figure 3.1 Hierarchy of a relational database

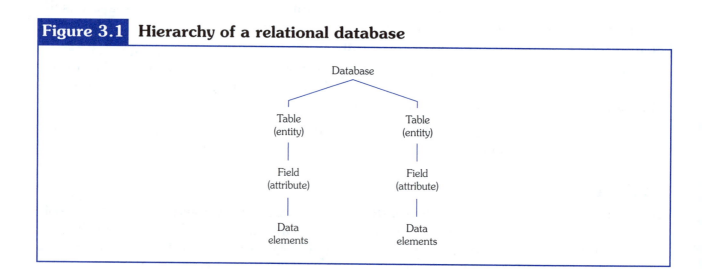

Figure 3.2 shows the ERD for the multiple tables in the compliance education database developed in Microsoft Access.

Figure 3.2 **Entity relationship diagram**

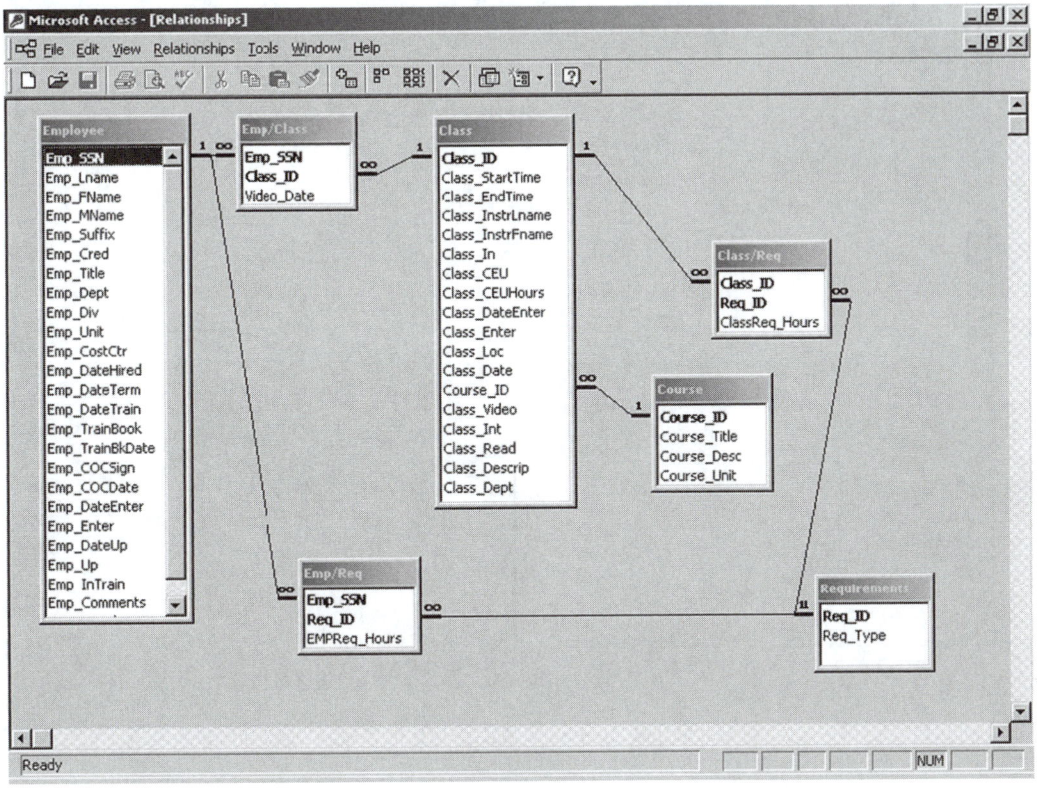

Data Dictionaries

A **data dictionary** is the equivalent of a detailed road map of the database. It is essential to ensuring consistent definitions of what data names mean and making sure that data are accurate. A good dictionary defines each data field or column according to the following information:

- Name of computer or software program that contains the data element
- Type of data in the field
- Length of data in the field
- Edits placed on the data field
- Values allowed to be placed in the data field
- A clear definition of each value (Sayles 2012,882–884).

Figure 3.3 shows a partial data dictionary for the "patient" table.

Figure 3.3 Partial data dictionary

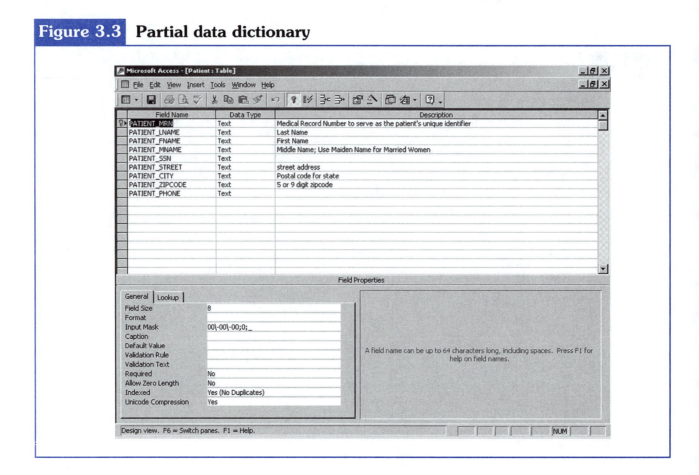

For additional information on data dictionaries, read the AHIMA practice brief "Guidelines for Developing a Data Dictionary."

Understanding database design requires various skills. Robert Campbell details 50 different skills in his article "Database Design: What HIM Professionals Need to Know." Campbell found through his research that the most highly ranked skill necessary for working with databases is fluency in the SQL command language. In the article, he also provides a solid discussion of the use of databases in the United States and a listing of references related to database skills, providing additional reading for those who are interested (Campbell 2004).

Structured Query Language (SQL)

Structured query language (SQL) is a flexible language that is commonly used to communicate with a relational database. It uses queries to retrieve data. If any of the data in the database satisfy the conditions of the query, SQL retrieves the information. For example, a query statement might ask the database to retrieve data for all of the patients with a length of stay greater than or equal to five days who received penicillin. SQL would display a list of patients where the conditions were satisfied.

SQL actually contains three languages. It is a data definition language (DDL), used to define a database or modify its structure; a data manipulation language (DML), used to enter, change, or extract data; and a data control language (DCL), used to protect the database from being corrupted and to provide security.

A simple **query** statement using the DML has three parts. The "select" statement is always first. This determines the label, or field name, of the data that is being retrieved. The next statement is always the "from" statement, telling the database which table is to be used. The last statement is the "where" statement, which lists the conditions that must be satisfied for the data to be included.

A simple query to retrieve all patients from Milwaukee from the "patient" table shown in figure 3.3 would look like this:

```
SELECT PATIENT_LNAME, PATIENT_FNAME
FROM PATIENT
WHERE PATIENT_CITY = 'Milwaukee'
```

When retrieving data from multiple tables in a database, a join function must be used to connect the tables together. In the example above, if information on the patient's insurance company was also required, the "insurance" table would be joined to the "patient" table using "PATIENT_MRN" for the primary and foreign key. The "from" statement would list both table names, separated by a comma. For example:

```
SELECT PATIENT_LNAME, PATIENT_FNAME
FROM PATIENT, INSURANCE
WHERE PATIENT_MRN = PATIENT_MRN
AND PATIENT_CITY = 'Milwaukee'
```

The Use of Statistical Software Packages

Use of the software to help in statistical analysis of large databases began in the mid-1960s and has grown to a multibillion-dollar business in the 21st century. These specialized software packages make the analysis process possible on even the largest databases. The two most popular software packages on the market today are **Statistical Analysis System (SAS)** and **Statistical Package for the Social Sciences (SPSS)**. The preference for one particular type of software may be made based on the formal education or individualized learning of the analyst. SPSS is primarily menu-driven software, but may be programmed using command lines. SAS is primarily a command line software tool and requires the analyst to have knowledge of both the statistical techniques as well as the command syntax to complete the analysis.

Statistical Analysis System (SAS)

SAS is a software package for data analytics that has ready-to-use programs for data manipulation, information storage and retrieval, statistics, and report writing.

It allows the user to bring together data from different platforms and data structures for analysis.

The SAS program communicates what you want to do in a sequence of statements executed in order on an SAS data set. The programs are created in two basic steps: the data (DATA) step and the procedure (PROC) step. The data step may be used to create a dataset or to create new variables within an existing dataset. The PROC step is used to run a statistical analysis procedure.

The following is a simple SAS program that converts miles to kilometers in a data step and prints the results with a procedure step:

```
DATA step:      DATA distance;
                Miles = 26.22;
                Kilometers =1.161 * Miles;
PROC step:      PROC PRINT DATA = distance;
                RUN;
```

The output resulting from the previous SAS statements is:

Obs	Miles	Kilometers
1	26.22	30.4414

Note that each SAS statement must end in a semicolon (Delwiche and Slaughter 2003, 6). The semi colon is a signal to the SAS program that the statement is complete. The SAS commands are not executed until a "run" statement is encountered.

SAS is an excellent tool for handling large datasets. Although SAS does include the ability to run procedures and manipulate data via a menu driven interface, it traditionally is used by writing command line code as in the example above.

Statistical Package for the Social Sciences (SPSS)

Statistical Package for the Social Sciences (SPSS) is a statistical package for data analytics and is known for its ability to mine text as well as data. Unlike SAS, SPSS is primarily implemented using menus and wizards that guide the user through the steps of the analysis. The software package is organized in a modular fashion, with various specialty packages working along with the base statistical software. Output from SPSS is presented in the later chapters in the context of each analytic technique.

Specialized Databases

Data analysts may be asked to develop and maintain separate databases or, more typically, a separate data warehouse, to perform quality reporting, such as a **Healthcare Effectiveness Data and Information Set (HEDIS)** or hospital quality measures for the Centers for Medicare and Medicaid Services (CMS). Quality reporting cannot normally be completed by exclusively using the data that is already coded for healthcare statistics and reimbursement, as described in chapter 2, but this coded data plays a large role. The programmer typically selects (via programming language) the denominator cases based on age, enrollment, or other service criteria as well as on event or diagnosis criteria. The numerator is determined programmatically (via programming language from transaction data) or by health record review, which could involve manual data entry. Further discussion of quality reporting can be found in chapter 9.

Data Reports

When external data are obtained and used to produce a report or solve a problem, always remember to cite the source of the data, including the year. In addition, any data report should include the date and time that the report was run, regardless of the type of data used.

Managing versions of data (version control) is especially important when data requests are being refined, or if report specifications change throughout the reporting process, or until a final version is obtained. Multiple copies of the same report without a run date and time can lead to confusion and complicate the data analysis process. As the data manipulation begins, it is advisable to maintain the data in the original form and make a copy to use for data manipulation.

The Role of Microsoft Excel in Data Analysis

Microsoft Office Excel, commonly called Excel, is a proprietary spreadsheet application written and distributed by Microsoft. It features calculations, extensive graphing tools, and pivot tables, and is overwhelmingly the dominant spreadsheet application. The cells are organized in rows and columns and contain data or formulas with relative or absolute references to other cells. Excel allows the user to define the appearance of spreadsheets (fonts, character attributes, and cell appearance) (Microsoft Office Online 2010).

Excel 2007/2010/2013 files have an .xlsx extension, and older files use the .xls extension. Excel spreadsheets can accept data from other programs using the comma-separated values (CSV) format and other text files. The CSV format is a delimited data format that has fields or columns separated by the comma character and records or rows separated by new lines (Microsoft SQL Server Developer Center 2008). Cells can be formatted to display text, numbers, currency, percentages, dates, and other types of data. Note that cells containing International Classification of Diseases, ninth revision, Clinical Modification (ICD-9-CM) diagnoses and procedure codes need to be formatted as text in the Excel spreadsheet, as Excel does not recognize the lead or trailing zeros in ICD-9-CM codes by default and treats them as numbers. If the numerical formatting is maintained and the lead zeros are removed, the codes no longer appear in a meaningful format. This formatting is especially important as data are imported from other programs.

A detailed presentation of the Microsoft Excel Data Analysis Toolpak may be found in appendix B.

The Role of Microsoft Excel in Graphical Display of Data

Tables and graphs are tools for depicting data. Tables show summarized data, and graphs are useful for presenting relationships in visual form.

Microsoft Excel creates tables as data are entered. Graphs are easily created using the graphing features of the program. As data are highlighted in the spreadsheet, Excel suggests the best type of graph to use in displaying the data.

Tables

A table groups data in rows and columns; this format is similar to what is used in a spreadsheet. These tables are the starting point for creating graphic display of data. This display provides visual clues to important information at a glance. Tables are commonly incorporated with their graphic representation to provide the details that may be necessary for some readers.

It can be helpful to design the table before obtaining the data. Each table should include a descriptive title, including the date range for the data, and columns with understandable headings. Row captions at the far left are called stubs. Stubs are especially useful when data will be displayed in subgroups such as monthly totals or subsections of a population.

The data should move from left to right, with totals at the far right, and top to bottom, with totals at the bottom. Data is found in a cell, or the intersection of a row and a column. All of the data in one row pertains to one item (a patient, a code, or a similar entry), and all of the data in one column pertains to the same variable for each item in the rows. The columns are the variables, and the observations are the rows.

The source of the data should always be listed at the bottom of the table in case readers want to research further.

Graphs

Graphs display the data contained in tables but in an easy to read and easy to understand pictorial version. Graphs help draw the eye to relationships between the data and to areas of greatest importance. Charts are easiest to read when the height of the graph is approximately three-fourths the length of the graph (Osborn 2006).

The title of the graph should match the table it refers to or be made using the same guidelines presented above. When several variables are included on the same graph, a legend, or key, should be used for their identification. The vertical axis should always start at zero. The x axis is read from the lowest value on the left to the highest on the right. The scale of values from the y axis extends from the lowest value at the bottom of the graph to the highest at the top. As with tables, the exact reference to an outside data source should be given (Horton 2011, 206–207).

Bar Graphs

Graphs can be simple and display one variable or more complex and display two or more variables. Figure 3.4 shows an example of a two-variable bar graph showing the number of admissions by both age and gender.

Figure 3.4 Two-variable bar graph

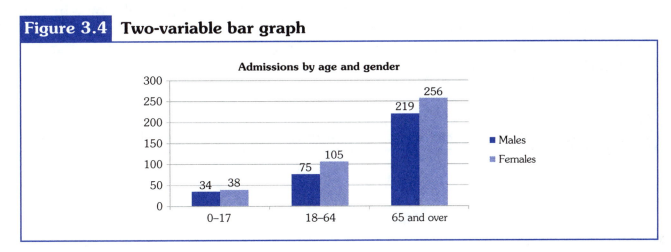

Line Graphs

Line graphs can also be referred to as run charts in the quality management field. Line graphs display time trends, percentages, and curves, such as the bell curves that will be discussed in chapter 9.

Pie Charts

Pie charts represent the data as component parts of the whole. The circle, or pie, is divided into sections that look like wedges or slices, each representing a percentage of the total. Therefore, data must be converted to percentages before the pie chart can be built. To emphasize the most important percentage, a pie slice can be highlighted or cut out of the pie. Figure 3.5 shows a pie chart with a cutout for the percentage of medicine admissions.

Figure 3.5 Pie chart with cutout section

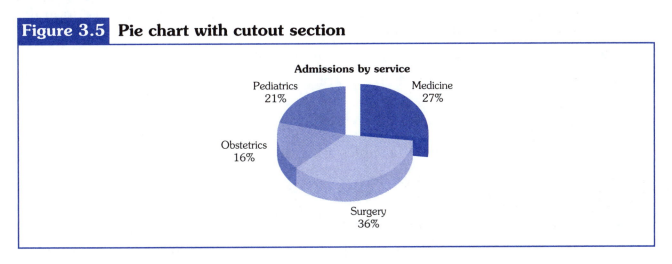

Scatter Diagrams

A scatter diagram, also called a scattergram or scatter plot, is a graph that is used to determine whether there is a correlation, or relationship, between two ratio or interval variables. Correlation will be discussed further in chapter 6.

Figure 3.6 shows a scatter diagram that depicts a positive linear relationship in a variable with two values. The variable is plotted based on the intersection of two values. The first few values in this scatter diagram are 1 and 1, 2 and 3, 3 and 2, and 4 and 5. The relationship is positive because an imaginary line moves from left to right on an ever-increasing slope.

Figure 3.6   Scatter diagram showing a positive linear relationship

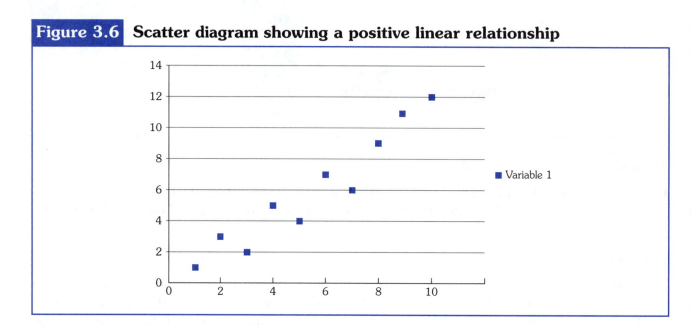

The Data Display Decision

The data analyst may be faced with the question of whether to use tables or graphs, and which graph is best to display the data. The answer most often depends upon the audience or the recipient of the report.

Tables have several advantages over graphs such as:

- Present more information than a graph
- Display the exact values
- Require less work to create

Graphs also have advantages over tables such as:

- Catch the attention of the reader
- Show trends easily
- Bring out facts or relationships that stimulate thinking

Many reports use a combination of tables, graphs, and narrative descriptions to tell the story of the data.

Review Questions

1. A scatterplot may be used to display the relationship between what data type(s)?
   a. Interval or ratio
   b. Qualitative
   c. Nominal
   d. Ordinal

2. A SAS statement always ends with what type of punctuation?
   a. .
   b. ,
   c. ;
   d. :

3. Which of the following keywords may be listed first in an SAS program?
   a. SET
   b. COUNT
   c. PROC
   d. SELECT

4. Which of the following keywords precedes the listing of variables to be returned from a SQL query?
   a. SELECT
   b. SET
   c. DATA
   d. BY

5. SPSS is a
   a. Statistical analysis software package
   b. Type of database
   c. Data warehouse
   d. Type of graph

6. What type of graph is most appropriate to display the average length of stay by hospital?
   a. Scatter graph
   b. Bar graph
   c. Pie graph
   d. Line graph

7. What type of graph is most appropriate to display the average length of stay by year?
   a. Bar graph
   b. Scatter graph
   c. Pie graph
   d. Line graph

8. A data dictionary is a:
   a. Definitions of each data field
   b. Listing of the tables included in a database
   c. Summary of the values of the data fields
   d. Graphical display of the structure of the database

9. Which of the following queries will provide a listing of patients who had services performed by Dr. X during 2007?
   a. SELECT PATIENT_LNAME, PATIENT_FNAME
       FROM PATIENT
       WHERE PHYSICIAN_NAME = 'X'
       AND ENC_DATE > '2006'
   b. SELECT PATIENT_LNAME, PATIENT_FNAME
       FROM PATIENT, ENCOUNTERS
       WHERE PATIENT_MRN = PATIENT_MRN
       AND PHYSICIAN_NAME = X
       AND ENC_DATE < '2008'
   c. SELECT PATIENT_LNAME, PATIENT_FNAME
       FROM PATIENT, ENCOUNTERS
       WHERE PATIENT_MRN = PATIENT_MRN
       AND PHYSICIAN_NAME = 'X'
       AND ENC_YEAR = '2007'
   d. SELECT PATIENT_LNAME, PATIENT_FNAME
       FROM PATIENT
       WHERE PHYSICIAN_NAME = 'X'
       AND ENC_YEAR = 2007

10. Consider the following data related to medication errors:

Dosage form	6%
Name confusion	13%
Communication	19%
Labeling	20%
Human factors	42%

Which of the following would be the best choice for the graphical display of the data?
   a. Line graph
   b. Bar graph
   c. Pie chart
   d. Data table

📖 References

AHIMA e-HIM Work Group on EHR Data Content. 2006. Guidelines for Developing a Data Dictionary. *Journal of AHIMA* 77(2): 64A-D.

Campbell, R.J. 2004. Database design: What HIM professionals need to know. *Perspectives in Health Information Management* 1:6 (August 2004).

Delwiche, L. and S. Slaughter. 2003. *The Little SAS® Book: A Primer*, 3rd ed. Cary, NC: SAS Institute Inc.

Horton, L.A. 2011. *Calculating and Reporting Healthcare Statistics*, 4th ed. Chicago: AHIMA.

Microsoft Office Online. Office Excel 2010 Product Overview. http://office.microsoft.com/en-us/excel/excel-2010-features-and-benefits-HA101806958.aspx

Microsoft SQL Server Developer Center. 2008. Exporting to a CSV File. http://msdn.microsoft.com/en-us/library/ms155919(v=SQL.100).aspx

Osborn, C.E. 2006. *Statistical Applications for Health Information Management*, 2nd ed. Sudbury, MA: Jones and Bartlett Publishers.

Sayles, N. 2012. *Health Information Management Technology: An Applied Approach*, 4th ed. Chicago: AHIMA.

Taylor, A.G. 2006. *SQL For Dummies*, 6th ed. Hoboken, NJ: Wiley Publishing Inc.

Analyzing Categorical Variables

KEY TERMS

Alpha level

Alternative hypothesis

Bell curve

Binomial variable

Chi-squared

Confidence interval

Confidence level

Contingency tables

Critical value

Frequency chart

Frequency distribution

Independent

Margin of error

Null hypothesis

One sample Z-test for proportions

P-value

Percentile rank

Pie chart

Rank

Standard error

Standard normal distribution

Test statistic

Two-sample Z-test for proportions

Type I error

Type II error

Categorical variables are data elements that represent categories and are either nominal or ordinal. The analysis of categorical variables requires a methodology that describes the membership in the categories and the patterns in relative proportion of the sample in each category. For this chapter, we will assume that the data is assigned to mutually exclusive and exhaustive categories. Mutually exclusive means that the categories cannot overlap. Exhaustive means that every subject will fit into a category. Another way to say mutually exclusive and exhaustive is to say that each subject is assigned to one and only one category.

Examples of categorical data in healthcare include: gender, discharge status, admission source or Medicare severity-adjusted diagnosis-related group (MS-DRG). A special case of a categorical variable is a binary variable. A binary variable has two values: yes or no. Most rates used in healthcare are based on binary variables. For instance, a mortality rate may be compiled by assigning a one for every patient that dies and a zero for every patient that does not die. The average of that binary variable is the mortality rate.

Descriptive Statistics

Frequency Distributions of Coded Data

The table used to display a **frequency distribution** can be used to display the various codes used and the number of times each code has been assigned. The frequency distributions form the starting point for data tables regarding diagnosis-related groups, ambulatory patient classification, Current Procedural Terminology (CPT) codes, relative value unit values, and bell curve displays, are subjects that will be discussed in upcoming chapters. In addition, frequency distributions of ICD-9-CM diagnosis codes and CPT codes can provide valuable information for the development of charge tickets, billing sheets, or superbills in physician offices. Table 4.1 shows an example of a frequency distribution of patient gender.

Table 4.1 Frequency table – patient gender

Gender	Count	Percent
Female	32	57%
Male	24	43%
Grand Total	**56**	**100%**

The distribution of the CPT codes for new patients billed by hospital outpatient departments during Calendar Year 2011 is displayed in table 4.2. This data was extracted from the CMS 2013 Final Rule data files (CMS 2012a):

Table 4.2 Frequency table – new office/outpatient visit CPT codes

HCPCS	Definition	Total Frequency	Percent
99201	Level 1 – Office or outpatient visit new	155,168	17%
99202	Level 2 – Office or outpatient visit new	172,459	18%
99203	Level 3 – Office or outpatient visit new	279,312	30%
99204	Level 4 – Office or outpatient visit new	219,398	24%
99205	Level 5 – Office or outpatient visit new	104,442	11%
Total		**930,779**	**100%**

Frequency charts are an excellent tool for displaying the distribution of categorical variables. In a frequency chart, the horizontal axis represents the categories and the vertical axis represents the count of the number of subjects in each category. Frequency charts are a special case of the bar charts presented in chapter 3. The frequency chart for the new office or outpatient visit CPT code distribution is displayed in figure 4.1.

Figure 4.1 **Frequency chart – new office/outpatient visit CPT codes**

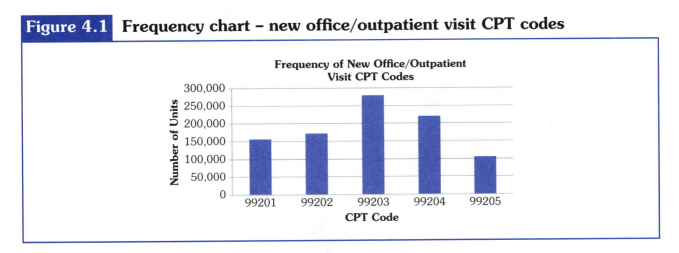

Notice that the axes of the frequency chart are both labeled so the reader will know immediately what the horizontal axis represents and what the height of the bars represents. The power of the frequency chart is that the pattern is more readily observed in the table format.

Categorical data may also be presented using a pie chart. A **pie chart** is a circular graph where the slices of the circle or pie represent the proportion of the subjects that are in each category. The pie chart for the new office visit CPT codes appears in figure 4.2.

Figure 4.2 **Pie chart – new office/outpatient visit CPT codes**

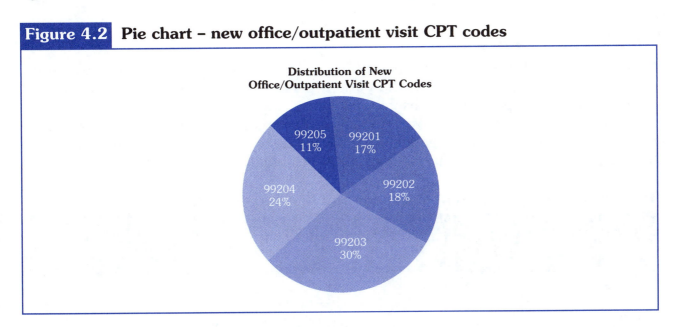

In this case, the pie chart does not convey the ordinal nature of the CPT codes. In other words, this set of CPT codes has an inherent order of level one through level five. That concept is lost when viewing this data as a pie chart. The frequency chart in figure 4.1 is a better representation of the CPT code data since the order on the horizontal axis does demonstrate the order of the codes in terms of level.

A pie chart is actually an excellent graph to use when presenting nominal data. The pie chart for the patient gender data from table 4.1 appears in figure 4.3. This clearly shows that the majority of the patients are male. Since there is not order to the gender designations, the pie chart is the appropriate graph to use in presenting the gender distribution. Selecting the correct graph for a particular set of data is sometimes difficult, but an analyst should always select a presentation that conveys meaning without misleading the reader.

Figure 4.3 **Pie chart – gender**

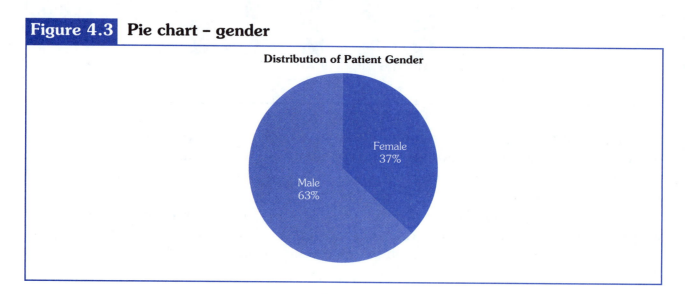

Contingency Tables

Contingency tables are a useful method for displaying the relationship between two categorical variables. Suppose in the patient gender example above, an indicator of whether or not the patient was discharged to their home was also collected. Table 4.3 shows a contingency table or cross tabulation of the patient gender and the discharged to home variable. This contingency table allows us to see that a larger proportion of female patients were sent home (20 out of 32) than males (14 out of 24).

Table 4.3 Contingency table of gender and discharged to home

Gender	Discharged Home		
	Home	Not Home	Row Total
Female	20	12	32
Male	10	14	24
Column Total	30	26	56

Contingency tables are often referred to by the number of rows and columns. Table 4.3 is a 2 × 2 (rows × columns) contingency table. The grand totals for the rows and columns are not counted and the title columns are not counted. The blanks in the body of the table that house the counts of subjects in each of the row and column categories are called cells. The number seven in the "male" x "not home" cell tells us that 14 male subjects were not sent home.

Rank

Rank denotes a value's position in a group relative to other values that have been organized in order of magnitude. Ranking is an excellent method of summarizing ordinal data. The statistic is not applicable to nominal data, since that type of data does not have an inherent order.

In addition to determining the rank of the value in a group, it can be helpful to divide the values into smaller parts to better understand the relationship of all values to each other. Data organized in order of magnitude can be divided into four equal parts, or quartiles. The first quartile stretches to the first 25 percent of the data, the second quartile from 25 percent to 50 percent of the data (median), and so on. In similar fashion, deciles represent data divided into 10 equal parts. The first decile corresponds to the 10th percentile and includes the first 10 percent of the values in the distribution.

The most commonly used division is percentiles, which separate the distribution into 100 equal parts. If a person scores at the 54th percentile, the score is greater than or equal to 54 percent of all the scores in the distribution. This is called **percentile rank**, and it helps the reader understand the relationship of the value to the remainder of the values in the distribution. Standardized academic and admissions test scores are often reported with percentile ranks along with raw scores so that students understand where they scored relative to their peers.

Inferential Statistics

Hypothesis Testing Basics

A contingency table summarizes the relationship between two categorical variables and allows the values to be compared. The table represents a descriptive statistical approach to characterizing the distribution of the subjects among the cells in the table. In the example in table 4.3, we observed that the proportion of female patients sent home was higher than the proportion of males sent home. An analyst may want to apply inferential statistics to determine if the proportion sent home is statistically different between the genders, or if the descriptive statistics observed might just be due to chance or random variation that can occur when drawing a sample from the larger population of patient. If there is indeed a gender difference in discharge destination, that may help target discharge planning programs. A hypothesis test is the inferential tool used to determine if there is a statistical difference in the genders.

In this first example of a hypothesis test, it is important to review some vocabulary. The first step in statistical hypothesis testing is defining the null and alternative hypotheses.

The **null hypothesis** is the status quo. In our contingency table example, the null hypothesis is that there is no relationship between the gender of the subject and whether or not they were discharged to home. The statistical term for no relationship for two variables is that they are **independent**. The **alternative hypothesis** is the complement of the null hypothesis and typically requires some action to be taken. In our example, the alternative hypothesis is that there is a significant relationship between gender and likelihood to be discharged home, or that the two variables are not independent.

The statistic used to test the hypothesis is called a **test statistic**. The test statistic is compared against the appropriate probability distribution to determine the probability of making an error when rejecting the null hypothesis. There are two types of errors in hypothesis testing: type I and type II. A **type I error** is made when the null hypothesis is rejected when it is actually true. A **type II error** is made when the null hypothesis is not rejected when it is actually false.

Type I error is set prior to performing a hypothesis test and is called the **alpha level** or simply the level of the test for short. The alpha level of a test should be set based on the risk or cost inherent in rejecting the null hypothesis when it is true. If the experiment involves the efficacy of a new treatment protocol, then the alpha level should be set low (one percent or five percent). If the experiment is to determine the favorite entrée at a local restaurant, then a much higher alpha level of 10 percent may be appropriate. The smallest alpha level for which the null hypothesis can be rejected based on the sample data collected is called the **p-value**.

Type II error depends on the statistical test used to test the hypothesis and the sample size. The statistical tests recommended in this text are the versions that minimize the type II error. The choice is somewhat in the control of the data analyst, but much less so than type I error. Type II error is also impacted by the sample size selected for the experiment. A larger sample size will decrease the level of type II errors. The proper selection of sample size and the impact of that choice on type II error will be discussed in a later chapter.

The steps in testing statistical hypotheses are as follows:

1. Determine the null and alternative hypotheses
2. Set the acceptable type I error or alpha level
3. Select the appropriate test statistic
4. Compare the test statistic to a critical value based on alpha and the distribution of the test statistic
5. Reject the null hypothesis if the calculated test statistic is more extreme than the critical value. If not, then do not reject the null hypothesis

Chi-squared Test of Independence

Chi-squared, represented by the symbol X^2 (where X is the Greek letter chi.), is a statistical test that is used to test for relationships between categorical variables. A chi-squared test may be generated by hand, but using computer software or an online statistical calculator is much easier. The first step in using any hypothesis testing procedure in statistics is to understand the null and alternative hypothesis to be tested.

For the chi-squared test, the null hypothesis is that there is no association between the categorical variables or that they are independent. The alternative hypothesis is that there is some relationship or association between the variables. In our gender versus discharged to home example, the null hypothesis is that the proportion of patients sent home is statistically the same for both genders. In viewing the cross tabulation in table 4.3, we can see that 20 out of 32 (63 percent) of the females were discharged to home, but only 10 out of 24 (42 percent) of the males were discharged to home. A chi-squared test may be used to determine if the results from this sample of patients can be generalized to conclude a difference in proportion sent home in the two genders.

In formulating the test statistic for the chi-squared test, we determine the expected number of patients per cell and compare that to the observed values in each of the cells. If patient gender and discharge destination were independent, then we would expect the proportion of patients in the home and not home categories to be the same for each gender. If the observed values are very different from the expected counts, then we can conclude that the null hypothesis is false and the two variables are not independent. The chi-squared test statistic will tell us the probability of observing the values if the null hypothesis is true. If that probability is small enough, then we may conclude that gender and discharged home or not home are related. The acceptable probability of making an error is set prior to running the statistical test and is called the alpha level of the test. For this example, we will set the alpha level to be five percent, or 0.05.

Table 4.4 Cell labeling for chi-squared test

Gender	Discharged Home	
	Home	Not Home
Female	A	B
Male	C	D

Using the cell labeling found in table 4.4, the expected cell frequencies for each cell may be calculated using the following formula:

$$Expected\ cell\ frequency = \frac{(row\ total) \times (column\ total)}{(grand\ total\ of\ all\ cells)}$$

Table 4.5 Calculation of expected cell frequencies

Gender	Discharged Home	
	Home	Not Home
Female	= (32*30)/56	= (32×26)/56
Male	= (24*30)/56	= (24*26)/56

Table 4.6 Expected cell frequencies

Gender	Discharged Home		
	Home	Not Home	Row Total
Female	17.1	14.9	32.0
Male	12.9	11.1	24.0
Column Total	30.0	26.0	56.0

Notice that the row and column totals for the expected frequencies in table 4.6 and the observed frequencies in table 4.3 is the same. It is the distribution of the values among the cells that are different. The chi-squared test statistic may now be calculated using the following formula:

$$X^2 = \sum_{i,j} \frac{(O_{ij} - E_{ij})^2}{E_{ij}}$$

Where O_{ij} is the observed frequency in the cell in row i and column j and E_{ij} is the expected cell frequency in row i and column j. Using the example data, the chi-squared statistic is as follows:

$$X^2 = \frac{(20-17.1)^2}{17.1} + \frac{(12-14.9)^2}{14.9} + \frac{(10-12.9)^2}{12.9} + \frac{(14-11.1)^2}{11.1} = 2.39$$

An extreme value for a test statistic is indicative of a statistically significant result. For the chi-squared test, the value of the test statistic should be compared to the chi-squared distribution with one degree of freedom to determine the probability of incorrectly rejecting the null hypothesis is less than our pre set alpha level of five percent. Table 4.7 includes the critical value values for common alpha levels used for a chi-squared test. A **critical value** is the value that a test statistic must be larger than to conclude statistical significance. The value is based on the alpha level of the test and the distribution of the test statistic if the null hypothesis is true.

The X^2 distribution is depending on the number of degrees of freedom in the experiment. When testing for independence of the rows and columns of a contingency table, the degrees of freedom are determined by multiplying the number of rows minus one times the number of columns minus one. In our example this is $(2 - 1) \times (2 - 1) = 1$. If the value of test statistic is greater than the critical value associated with the degrees of freedom and alpha level for our situation, then the null hypothesis should be rejected. The test statistic is 2.39. This value is not greater than 3.841, therefore, we do not reject the null hypothesis and conclude that our sample does not represent statistical evidence that gender and discharge status home are not independent.

Table 4.7 Chi-squared with one degree of freedom critical values

Alpha level	X^2 Critical Value (df = 1)
0.1	2.706
0.05	3.841
0.025	5.024
0.01	6.635
0.005	7.879

In testing a hypothesis using statistical inference, the decision is to reject or not reject the null hypothesis at the preset alpha level. The words used to express the conclusion of a hypothesis test are often confusing to analysts when they begin using statistical tests to generalize the results of their sample. It typically involves phrasing conclusions as double-negatives such as, "There is no evidence that two variables are not independent." You are not concluding that the two variables are independent, just that there is no evidence that they are not independent.

Example 4.1 – Chi-squared test of independence

Employees at a large healthcare facility were randomly asked whether they smoked and whether they had parents who smoked. The results of the 150 employees sampled are as follows:

	Parents who smoke	Parents who do not smoke
Employee smokes	45	25
Employee does not smoke	30	50

The data in this table suggest that those employees with parents who did not smoke were likelier not to smoke (50 vs. 25) than were those employees with parents who smoked (30 vs. 45). From this sample alone, there appears to be a relationship between smoking and having parents who smoke. A chi-squared test may be used to test the null hypothesis that an employee's smoking status and their parents' smoking status are independent. This is where a chi-squared test can help determine whether the relationship is significant. Prior to testing the hypothesis, the alpha level is set to five percent. Recall the formula for the chi-squared test:

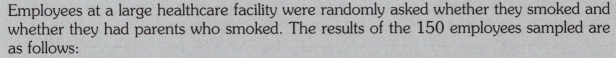

$$X^2 = \sum_{i,j} \frac{(O_{ij} - E_{ij})^2}{E_{ij}}$$

(continued)

Example 4.1 – Chi-squared test of independence (*continued*)

Step 1: Calculate the expected cell values

	Parents who smoke	Parents who do not smoke
Employee smokes	= [(45 + 25) × (45 + 30)]/150	= [(45 + 25) × (25 + 50)]/150
Employee does not smoke	= [(30 + 50) × (45 + 30)]/150	= [(30 + 50) × (25 + 50)]/150

	Parents who smoke	Parents who do not smoke
Employee smokes	35	35
Employee does not smoke	40	40

Step 2: Calculate the test statistic

$$X^2 = \frac{(45-35)^2}{35} + \frac{(25-35)^2}{35} + \frac{(30-40)^2}{40} + \frac{(50-40)^2}{40} = 10.71$$

Step 3: Determine cutoff from chi-square distribution with 1 degree of freedom and alpha level 0.05 from table 4.7.

Step 4: If test statistic value is greater than cutoff, then reject the null hypothesis. Since 10.71 > 3.841, we reject the null hypothesis and conclude that the employee's smoking status and their parent's smoking status are not independent.

In example 4.1, the null hypothesis of independence of the employee's and parent's smoking status was rejected at the 0.05 alpha level. Notice that the value of the chi-squared test statistic, 10.71, is larger than all of the values found in table 4.7. This means that the null hypothesis would be rejected even if the level or type I error rate was set to 0.005 or 0.5 percent. The smallest value of type I error for which the null hypothesis can be rejected is called the **p-value**. The p-value for an hypothesis test is often reported so that the reader can make the determination of whether or not the error rate is acceptable. In example 4.1, the p-value is less than 0.5 percent. If the reader is willing to be wrong less than 0.5 percent of the time, then they may reject the null hypothesis. Note that if a p-value is very small it is reported as "less than" the smallest value available in a table or in the computer output. A p-value is never reported as a zero.

Rates and Proportions

Rates and proportions are commonly found in healthcare data. Mortality, infection, and complication rates are tracked quality and outcomes measures. Many examples may be found on common healthcare data sites. CMS releases many of the indicators on their Hospital Compare website in the form of rates (see online appendix G). Figure 4.4 shows the rates for effective care of pneumonia patients for one hospital. These rates are reported to CMS as part of the value purchasing program and released publicly on a quarterly basis.

Figure 4.4	**CMS Hospital Compare pneumonia care rates (CMS)**
Pneumonia patients whose initial emergency room blood culture was performed prior to the administration of the first hospital dose of antibiotics ***Higher*** *percentages are better*	99%
Pneumonia patients given the most appropriate initial antibiotic(s) ***Higher*** *percentages are better*	95%

Source: CMS 2012.

When analyzing rates, the analyst must understand the definition of the numerator and denominator. The numerator of the rate is the count of subjects that meet the criteria to be measured. The denominator of the rate is the number of subjects that could meet the criteria. For example, if the inpatient mortality rate for congestive heart failure (CHF) is five percent at a local hospital we know that five percent of the patients admitted for CHF died in the hospital. The numerator is the number of patients admitted for CHF that died while in the hospital in the sample and the denominator is the number of patients admitted for CHF in the sample. A careful definition of the numerator and denominator is the key to creating rates that are reproducible and comparable across time.

The rates that CMS uses in Hospital Compare include documentation that carefully describes which patients should be included and excluded from the numerator and denominator to ensure that rates are comparable across facilities. For instance, the pneumonia indicators displayed in figure 4.4 both exclude patients with a diagnosis of cystic fibrosis and those with a length of stay greater than 120 days (CMS 2012b).

Descriptive Statistics

If the data used to compile a rate is thought of as a binary variable as having two values for each subject: one if the attribute is true and zero if it is not, then a rate is actually the average of those values. See example 4.2 for a demonstration.

Example 4.2 – Rate as an average

Suppose a sample of 10 employees is selected to estimate the compliance rate for obtaining a flu vaccine prior to the start of flu season. The analyst records a one in the data table if the employee had a vaccine and a zero if they did not. The data collected appears in the table below.

Employee	Vaccine? (1 = yes; 0 = no)
1	1
2	1
3	0
4	1
5	1
6	0
7	0
8	1
9	1
10	1
Average	0.7

Out of the 10 employees surveyed, seven received the flu vaccine. This results a rate of 0.7 or 70 percent. The value 0.7 is also the average of seven ones and three zeros. This strategy of recording rates as a series of binary (zero or one) value useful when using spreadsheet programs to calculate rates. Try this example using Excel.

If the rate for an event is rare, it may be reported as a count out of 1,000 or even 10,000. A percentage may be thought of as a rate out of 100. Reporting values such as 0.5 percent or 0.005 percent are difficult for the reader to interpret. Instead, rates for events that are rare are reported as 5 per 1,000 or 5 per 100,000. For example, the National Cancer Institute (NCI) Surveillance Epidemiology and End Results (SEER) database reports cancer rates in this manner (National Cancer Institute 2012). Figure 4.5 in an example of the reporting of a rare event. The age adjusted incident rate for lung and bronchus cancer is 62.6 per 100,000 per year or 0.0626 percent. The "per 100,000" statistic is much easier to interpret and understand than stating the rate as 62.6 hundredths of a percent.

In statistics, a variable that has two values and each independent trial or subject has the same probability of success is called a **binomial variable**. In example 4.2, an

Figure 4.5 **Lung and bronchus cancer rates from SEER database**

The age-adjusted incidence rate was 62.6 per 100,000 men and women per year. These rates are based on cases diagnosed in 2005-2009 from 18 SEER geographic areas.

Incidence Rates by Race

Race/Ethnicity	Male	Female
All Races	76.4 per 100,000 men	52.7 per 100,000 women
White	76.4 per 100,000 men	55.1 per 100,000 women
Black	99.9 per 100,000 men	52.6 per 100,000 women
Asian/Pacific Islander	52.2 per 100,000 men	28.8 per 100,000 women
American Indian/Alaska Native	51.9 per 100,000 men	37.4 per 100,000 women
Hispanic	40.5 per 100,000 men	25.8 per 100,000 women

Source: National Cancer Institute, 2012.

employee that obtained a flu vaccine might be considered a success. If we were to pick an employee at random, each would have a probability of 0.7 or 70 percent of having obtained a flu vaccine. The properties of the binomial distribution form the basis for the inferential statistics that may be used in studying rates and proportions. A full discussion of binomial variables and their distribution is beyond the scope of this text, but understanding the basis of the inferential statistics is important.

Inferential Statistics

One-sample Z-test for proportions

After calculating a rate, the next step is typically to compare that rate to some standard. In example 4.2, the flu vaccine compliance rate for employees was estimated to be 70 percent based on the sample of 10 percent. If the company goal was 85 percent compliance, does the rate in the sample represent a real difference from the goal or could that difference be due to random variation or bad luck in drawing the sample? A hypothesis test may be used to compare the observed compliance rate to the standard. The null hypothesis is that the population of interest is equal to the standard and the alternative hypothesis is that the population proportion is not equal to the standard (p_0). A one-sided hypothesis test may also be completed by defining the null hypothesis to be that the population proportion is less than (greater than) or equal to the standard and the alternative hypothesis as the converse H_0.

For a two-sided hypothesis test, where H_0 is the null hypothesis and H_a is the alternative hypothesis.

$H_0: p = p_0$

$H_a: p \neq p_0$

For a one-sided hypothesis test, where H_0 is the null hypothesis and H_a is the alternative hypothesis.

$H_0: p \leq p_0$
$H_a: p > p_0$
or
$H_0: p \geq p_0$
$H_a: p < p_0$

The steps in testing this hypothesis are the same as used in the chi-squared test:

1. Determine the null and alternative hypotheses
2. Set the acceptable type I error or alpha level
3. Select the appropriate test statistic
4. Compare the test statistic to a critical value based on alpha and the distribution of the test statistic
5. Reject the null hypothesis if the calculated test statistic is more extreme than the critical value. If not, then do not reject the null hypothesis

The test statistic used to compare a proportion to a standard is called the **one sample Z-test for proportions**. The formula for this test is:

$$Z = \frac{p - p_o}{\sqrt{p_o \times (1 - p_o) / n}}$$

Where p_o is the proportion value in the null hypothesis, p is the observed sample proportion and n is the sample size. The value of the test statistic, Z, is compared against critical values from the standard normal distribution for the acceptable level of type I error to determine if the null hypothesis should be rejected or not. The normal distribution is sometimes referred to as the **bell curve** because of its shape (see figure 4.6). The **standard normal distribution** is a bell shaped curve with a mean of zero and standard deviation of one.

Figure 4.6 **Standard normal distribution**

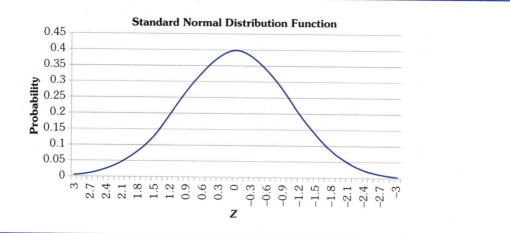

The critical values for common alpha levels may be found in table 4.8. A full standard normal distribution table may be found in many statistical texts or on-line.

Table 4.8 Common standard normal distribution critical values

Alpha level	Standard Normal Critical Value
0.1	1.282
0.05	1.645
0.025	1.960
0.01	2.326
0.005	2.576

Example 4.3 – One sample Z-test for proportions

Suppose the goal flu vaccine rate for a company is 85 percent. An analyst collected the compliance rates for a sample of 10 employees as presented in example 4.2. Use the sample data to determine if the company is meeting its compliance rate goal if the leaders are willing to accept a five percent chance of making the incorrect conclusion.

Since the analyst will be using sample data to make a conclusion about the population of company employees, this is an application of statistical inference. Specifically, the analyst can use the one sample Z-test for proportions to determine if the sample provides enough evidence to conclude that the vaccine compliance rate is different from the goal. The hypothesis steps are listed below:

1. Determine the null and alternative hypotheses:
   Null hypothesis (H_o): p = 85 percent or 0.85
   Alternative hypothesis (H_a): $p \neq 0.85$
2. Set the acceptable type I error or alpha level
   The company leaders are willing to accept a five percent error rate. Alpha = 0.05
3. Select the appropriate test statistic
   Z is the appropriate test statistic
4. Compare the test statistic to a critical value based on alpha and the distribution of the test statistic

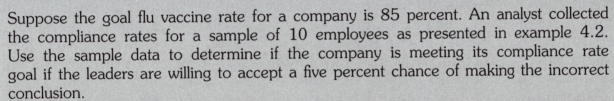

$$Z = \frac{0.70 - 0.85}{\sqrt{0.85 \times (1 - 0.85)/10}} = \frac{-.15}{0.11} = -1.36$$

(continued)

Example 4.3 – One sample Z-test for proportions (*continued*)

5. Reject the null hypothesis if the calculated test statistic is more extreme than the critical value. If not, then do not reject the null hypothesis

Since H_a is a two sided alternative ($\neq$) we select the critical value associated with the alpha level divided by two. We want to protect against both higher and lower alternatives. We reject H_o if $Z > 1.960$ or $Z < -1.960$. $Z = -1.36$ is not less than -1.960, therefore do not reject the null hypothesis.

The conclusion here is that the 70 percent rate observed in the sample of 10 employees is not far enough away from the goal of 85 percent to conclude that the observed rate is statistically different from the goal. The null hypothesis is not rejected.

Example 4.3 demonstrates why it is important to perform statistical tests prior to making a generalization from a sample to the population. The observed compliance rate of 70 percent may appear to be very different from the goal, but not "different enough" considering the error rate deemed acceptable by company leadership in making the conclusion. Examining the structure of the test statistic, Z, can help us understand why the null hypothesis was not rejected in this example. Notice that the numerator of the test statistic is the difference between the observed and null hypothesis rate. Large differences between the observed and null hypothesis rates will yield a larger test statistic and therefore a value that is more likely to result in rejecting the null hypothesis. The denominator of the test statistic includes both the null hypothesis rate and the sample size. Notice that if both the observed and null hypothesis rates stay constant and we change the sample size, the value of test statistic will increase. If we use a sample size of 30 with the same observed and null hypothesis values, then the value of Z is -2.30. This value is less than -1.960 and would result in rejecting the null hypothesis and concluding that the compliance rate is lower than the goal. The larger sample size provides stronger evidence against the null hypothesis. It makes intuitive sense that a larger sample size tells us more about the population. The formal statistical test allows the analyst to determine if the sample is giving enough evidence to reject the null hypothesis at the acceptable error level, given both the difference between the observed and null values as well as the sample size.

Confidence Interval for Proportions

In addition to testing the hypothesis that a proportion is different from a standard or goal value, an analyst may wish to formulate a range of reasonable values for the population proportion based on the sample values. This is commonplace in political surveys where a sample of voters is asked their opinions of Congress or the President, and the results are reported as a proportion or percentage plus or minus a margin of error. The margin of error is actually a form of statistical inference called a **confidence interval**. A confidence interval may be calculated so that it has a pre set probability of containing the population proportion. That probability is called the **confidence**

level and is the probability that the confidence interval contains the true population value of the proportion. The confidence interval is centered at the point estimate of the proportion plus or minus a margin of error that depends on a cutoff similar to the one defined in the one-sample Z-test for proportions. The formula for the confidence interval for a population proportion is:

$$p \pm (critical\ value\ for\ confidence\ level) \times \sqrt{\frac{p \times (1-p)}{n}}$$

In this formula, p is the sample proportion and n is the sample size. The critical value for the confidence level is found by taking (one minus the confidence level) divided by two. If we wish to formulate a 95 percent confidence interval, then the critical value is $(1 - 0.95)/2 = 0.025$.

Example 4.4 – Confidence interval for proportion

Suppose we wish to calculate a 95 percent confidence interval for the flu vaccine compliance rate based on the data presented in example 4.2. In that example, $p = 0.70$ and $n = 10$. The critical value is the value in table 4.7 associated with an alpha level of $(1-0.95)/2 = 0.025$.

$$0.70 \pm 1.96 \times \sqrt{\frac{0.70 \times (1-0.70)}{10}}$$

$$0.70 \pm 0.28$$
$$(0.42, 0.98)$$

The results: We are 95 percent sure that the interval from 0.42 to 0.98 contains the true population proportion of flu vaccine compliance. Another way to state the result is that we are 95 percent sure that the company compliance rate is 70 percent plus or minus 28 percent.

In example 4.4 the confidence interval is very wide. The width of the confidence interval is a measure of the precision of the point estimate of the proportion and is sometimes referred to as the **margin of error**. A narrow confidence interval is more precise than a wider confidence interval. Notice from the formula that the width of the confidence interval is the function of three variables: confidence level, sample size, and sample proportion. The analyst has control over the first two variables. A sample size will be discussed in a later chapter. Increasing the confidence level and leaving the other two components constant will result in a wider confidence interval. Often precision and confidence are a compromise based on budgetary constraints.

Two-sample Z-Test for Proportions

An analyst may be asked to compare the rates in two populations such as the mortality rates at two hospitals or the surgical site infection rate in two different units of a hospital. Hypotheses regarding two proportions may be tested using the **two-sample Z-test for proportions**. The null hypothesis in this case is that the two population proportions are equal. The alternative hypothesis may be single sided ($p_1 > p_2$ or $p_1 < p_2$) or two sided ($p_1 \neq p_2$).

For a two-sided hypothesis test:

$$H_0: p_1 = p_2$$
$$H_a: p_1 \neq p_2$$

For a one-sided hypothesis test:

$$H_0: p_1 \leq p_2$$
$$H_a: p_1 > p_2$$

or

$$H_0: p_1 \geq p_2$$
$$H_a: p_1 < p_2$$

The steps in testing such hypotheses follow the same five-step process outlined earlier. The formula for the test statistic is as follows:

$$Z = \frac{p_1 - p_2}{\sqrt{p \times (1 - p) \times \left[\dfrac{1}{n_1} + \dfrac{1}{n_2}\right]}}$$

$$where\ p = \frac{p_1 \times n_1 + p_2 \times n_2}{(n_1 + n_2)}$$

Where p_1 is the proportion from sample one, p_2 is the proportion from sample two, n_1 is the sample size from sample one and n_2 is the sample size from sample two. The test statistic in this case is more complex because it involves statistics derived from two samples. The denominator of Z is the **standard error** of the proportion pooled across the two samples. The standard error is a measure of the precision of the estimate of the proportions. It is a function of the standard deviation of the test statistic and the sample sizes. Notice that the formula is similar to the one-sample version. A large test statistic value may occur if the difference between the two sample proportions is large since that difference is in the numerator of the formula. A large sample size (n_1 and n_2) will result in a smaller denominator and a larger test statistic for any particular value of p_1 and p_2. These are important observations about the structure of the test statistic that will allow a better understanding of the influence of sample size selection in later chapters.

Example 4.5 – Comparing two proportions

Note: Data for this example comes from the Agency for Healthcare Research and Quality (AHRQ) Healthcare Cost and Utilization Project Network or HCUPnet (http://hcupnet.ahrq.gov/). The data collected by AHRQ for inclusion in HCUPnet is based on a combination of sample and complete data from selected states which require advanced analytic methods. For this example, we will assume that the data was collected via a random sample of patients throughout the country.

The MS-DRG system is designed so that patients with similar resource utilization are grouped together. A researcher wishes to investigate whether or not the inpatient mortality rates are different for heart failure and shock patients with major complications and comorbidities (MCC) versus those with no complications or comorbidities. Test the hypothesis that the mortality rates are the same for the two MS-DRGs below at the 0.05 level.

Outcomes for multiple specific diagnoses

Diagnosis Related Group and name		Total number of discharges	In-hospital deaths
291	Heart failure & shock w mcc	360,972	19,670 (5.45%)
293	Heart failure & shock w/o cc/mcc	197,734	2,148 (1.09%)

1. Determine the null and alternative hypotheses:

    $H_o: p_1 = p_2$ or $p_1 - p_2 = 0$

    $H_a: p_1 \neq p_2$ or $p_1 - p_2 \neq 0$

2. Set the acceptable type I error or alpha level

    Alpha = 0.05

3. Select the appropriate test statistic

    Z is the appropriate test statistic

4. Compare the test statistic to a critical value based on alpha and the distribution of the test statistic

$$p = \frac{0.0545 \times 360972 + 0.0109 \times 197734}{(360972 + 197734)} = \frac{21818}{558706} = 0.039$$

$$Z = \frac{0.0545 - 0.0109}{\sqrt{0.039 \times (1 - 0.039) \times \left[\frac{1}{360972} + \frac{1}{197734}\right]}} = 80.5$$

(continued)

Example 4.5 – Comparing two proportions (*continued*)

5. Reject the null hypothesis if the calculated test statistic is more extreme than the critical value. If not, then do not reject the null hypothesis

Since H_a is a two sided alternative ($\neq$), we reject H_o if $Z > 1.960$ or $Z < -1.960$. $Z = 80.5$ is greater than 1.64, therefore reject the null hypothesis and conclude that the mortality rate for patients assigned to MS-DRG 291 is significantly higher than that of patients assigned to MS-DRG 293.

✔ Review Questions

1. Which of the following variables should be summarized using a frequency distribution?
   a. Charge per case
   b. Diastolic blood pressure
   c. CPT codes
   d. Red blood cell count

2. Contingency tables may be used to:
   a. Describe the relationship between two interval variables
   b. Tabulate the number of subjects in a category
   c. Summarize continuous variables
   d. Display the relationship between two categorical variables

3. If an analyst collects data to determine if the mortality rate at her facility is different from the state average p_s, what are the appropriate null and alternative hypotheses?
   a. $H_o: p = p_s$ vs $H_A: p \neq p_s$
   b. $H_o: p \neq p_s$ vs $H_A: p = p_s$
   c. $H_o: p = p_s$ vs $H_A: p > p_s$
   d. $H_o: p \geq p_s$ vs $H_A: p < p_s$

4. In hypothesis testing, a type I error is:
   a. The probability of correctly accepting the null hypothesis
   b. The probability of incorrectly rejecting the null hypothesis
   c. The probability of incorrectly accepting the null hypothesis
   d. The probability of incorrectly rejecting the alternative hypothesis

5. A *p*-value is:
   a. The smallest type I error for which the null hypothesis will be rejected
   b. The estimated proportion
   c. The same as the alpha level
   d. The power of a test

6. If a chi-squared test statistic generated from a 2 × 2 contingency table is equal to 4.25 and the analyst is willing to accept an alpha level of five percent, what conclusion should be reported (using table 4.7)?
   a. Reject the null hypothesis and conclude that there is a relationship between the two variables
   b. Accept the null hypothesis and conclude there is not a relationship between the two variables
   c. Reject the alternative hypothesis and conclude there is not a relationship between the two variables
   d. Not enough information to make a conclusion

7. An analyst performed a hypothesis test and rejected the null hypothesis at an alpha level of 0.01. Based on that information, which of the following statements is true?
   a. The null hypothesis would be rejected at the 0.05 level
   b. The null hypothesis would not be rejected at the 0.05 level
   c. The null hypothesis would be rejected at all alpha levels
   d. Not enough information to determine if statements are true

8. An analyst wishes to compare the proportion of patients receiving take home supplies upon discharge from two units of the hospital. He draws a sample of 25 patients from two units of the hospital and finds that 10 patients discharged from Unit A received take home supplies and 15 patients from Unit B received take home supplies. What statistical tool should be used to determine if the two proportions are different?
   a. Confidence interval
   b. Frequency table
   c. One-sample Z-test for proportions
   d. Two-sample Z-test for proportions

9. The alpha level is:
   a. Always 0.05
   b. Based on the context of the analysis
   c. Set after the analysis is complete
   d. Never less than 0.01

10. A binomial variable:
   a. Is continuous variable
   b. A variable with two values
   c. A standardized variable
   d. Has a normal distribution

📖 References

Agency for Healthcare Research and Quality Healthcare Cost and Utilization Project Network. 2010. Outcomes for specific multiple diagnoses. http://hcupnet.ahrq.gov/

Centers for Medicare and Medicaid Services. 2012a. Details for Regulation No.: CMS-1589-FC. http://www.cms.gov/Medicare/Medicare-Fee-for-Service-Payment/HospitalOutpatientPPS/Hospital-Outpatient-Regulations-and-Notices-Items/CMS-1589-FC.html

Centers for Medicare and Medicaid Services. 2012b. Hospital Compare. http://www.medicare.gov/hospitalcompare/

National Cancer Institute. 2012. National Cancer Institute. http://seer.cancer.gov/statfacts/html/lungb.html

Analyzing Continuous Variables

KEY TERMS

Analysis of variance (ANOVA)

Balanced design

Levene's test

Mean

Measures of central tendency

Median

Mode

One-sample t-test

Paired t-test

Standard deviation

Standard error of the sample mean

Tukey Honest Significant Difference (HSD) Test

Two-sample t-test

Variance

Descriptive Statistics

Continuous variables include those measured on interval and ratio scales. Common continuous variables found in healthcare include: length of stay, wait times, charges, and laboratory test values. Descriptive statistics are used to summarize the center and shape of the distribution of a continuous variable. These are the two attributes of the data that are most important to end users:

"What is the typical value?" and "How spread out are the values?"

Measures of Central Tendency

In summarizing data, it is often useful to have a single typical value that is representative of the entire collection of data or specific population. Such numbers are customarily referred to as **measures of central tendency**. Three measures of central tendency are frequently used: mean, median, and mode. Each measure has advantages and disadvantages in describing a typical value.

The **mean** is the arithmetic average. It is computed by dividing the sum of all the values by the total number of values. The mean is the most common measure of central tendency and is the basis for a large proportion of statistical tests. The disadvantage of the mean is its sensitivity to extreme values, called outliers, which may bias its representation of the typical value of a set of numbers. The symbol for the mean is the letter x with a bar over the top. This is pronounced "x bar" in some settings. The mean is calculated by adding up the values and dividing by the number of values. The formal formula for the mean appears below:

$$\bar{x} = \frac{\sum_{i=1}^{n} x_i}{n} = \frac{x_1 + x_2 + \ldots + x_n}{n}$$

The mean is appropriate to use with data that is measured on an interval and ratio scale. The mean should not be used to summarize nominal or ordinal data. For example, favorite color is an example of nominal data. Even if numeric values were assigned to the various colors, taking the mean of those values would not provide any useful information.

Example 5.1

Suppose an ASC administrator wishes to measure the typical time a patient must wait from arrival at the center to being taken back for preparation for their procedure. She collects a sample of 10 patient wait times in minutes: 8, 15, 21, 4, 7, 11, 9, 5, 8, 10. What descriptive statistic should be used? Calculate the value.

Since time is a quantitative data element that is measured on a ratio scale, the mean is a valid measure of typical wait time.

$$\bar{x} = \frac{8 + 15 + 21 + 4 + 7 + 11 + 9 + 5 + 8 + 10}{10}$$

$$\bar{x} = \frac{98}{10} = 9.8 \text{ minutes}$$

The mean is sometimes applied to ordinal data in the field, but this is not best practice. As an example, consider a patient severity scale with four categories: typical, mild severity, moderate severity, major severity. An analyst recodes the severity scale data to 0, 1, 2, 3. Using the mean to describe the severity of the typical patient assumes that the difference between a typical and mildly severe patient is the same as the difference between a moderate and major severity patient. If that is the case, then the scale is actually an interval scale and the mean is an appropriate descriptive statistic. If that is not the case, then the mean is not measuring the typical severity level and may be providing misleading information to the end user.

The **median** is the midpoint (center) of the distribution of values, or the point above and below which 50 percent of the values fall. The median value is obtained by arranging the numerical observations in ascending or descending order and then determining the value in the middle of the array. If there is an even number of values, the median is a point halfway between the two middle values. This measure is not affected by extreme values. The steps to calculate the median are as follows:

1. Order the data values from smallest to largest
2. Count the number of values (n)
3. The median is:
    a. If n is an odd number, the median is the $\frac{n+1}{2}^{th}$ value.
    b. If n is an even number, the median is the average of the $\frac{n}{2}^{th}$ and the $(\frac{n}{2}+1)^{th}$ value.

Example 5.2

Suppose the ASC administrator from example 5.1 wishes to use the median to describe the wait time for the typical patient. Calculate the median of the 10 wait times 8, 15, 21, 4, 7, 11, 9, 5, 8, 10.

1. Order the values: 4, 5, 7, 8, 8, 9, 10, 11, 15, 21
2. $n = 10$
3. Since n is even, average the 5th and 6th values
4. Median $= \frac{8+9}{2} = 8.5$ minutes

Example 5.3

Suppose the ASC administrator from example 5.1 wishes to use the median to describe the wait time for the typical patient. Calculate the median and mean of the 11 wait times 8, 15, 21, 4, 7, 11, 9, 5, 8, 10, 45.

1. Order the values: 4, 5, 7, 8, 8, 9, 10, 11, 15, 21, 45
2. $n = 11$
3. Since n is odd, the median is the $(n + 1)/2$ value
4. Median $= 9$ minutes and Mean $= 13$ minutes

The mean and the median are both appropriate choices for describing the center of the distribution of interval, or ratio scaled data. The choice of which statistic to use is based on the presence or absence of extreme values in the data. The mean tends to be pulled toward extreme values while the median is not. Since the median has this property, it is described as a robust measure of central tendency, meaning that it is robust with respect to outliers, or that it is not as influenced by outliers as the mean. Example 5.3 illustrates this property of the median. Notice that the addition of the extreme value of 45 minutes has little impact of the median (8.5 minutes to 9.0 minutes), but has a significant impact on the mean (9.8 minutes to 13.0 minutes).

The mean is essentially pulled toward the extreme value, while the median is not. In this case, the median provides a better estimate of the typical patient wait time.

Mode is the third commonly used measure of central tendency and is the value that occurs most frequently in the data. This measure is rarely used as a measure of central tendency for continuous variables because it may not be unique. If multiple values all appear with the same frequency, each is a mode. In continuous data, it would not be unusual for all of the observations to have different values and therefore the entire sample of values may be the mode. The mode is typically used to determine the most frequent value in nominal and ordinal type data.

Measures of Variation

In addition to measuring the center of a distribution, we often need to have some measure of how spread out the distribution is. In other words, if an average charge for cataract surgery is $3,000 and we find that the values ranged from $1,500 to $7,500, then we would be less apt to depend on that measure to inform patients how much their procedure may cost than if the range was from $2,500 to $3,500. The most common measures of variation are range, variance, and standard deviation. They show how widely the observations are spread out around the measure of central tendency.

Range

The range is the simplest measure of spread. It indicates the difference between the largest and smallest values in a sample. Range has the advantage of being easy to compute, but is significantly affected by extreme values. Therefore, more informative measures of variation are variance and standard deviation. Using the data in example 5.2, the maximum wait time is 21 and the minimum wait time is 8. The range is then the maximum minus the minimum or 21 − 8 = 13.

Variance and Standard Deviation

The **variance** of a variable is the average of the squared standard deviations from the mean. The **standard deviation (sd)** is the square root of the variance. The units of analysis of the standard deviation is the same as the the units of the sample data. For example, the data in example 5.1 is measured in minutes. The unit of analysis of the variance of wait times is minutes squared. That is not very easy to interpret. Instead, the standard deviation or square root of the variance is often reported since it is measured in minutes. If the variance and standard deviation are small, there is less dispersion around the mean. If they are large, there is greater dispersion around the mean. The formula for the sample variance is:

$$s^2 = \frac{\sum_{i=1}^{n}(x_i - \bar{x})^2}{n-1}$$

The order of operations is important in calculating the sample variance. If the steps are not followed carefully, the value will be incorrect:

1. Calculate the sample mean
2. Calculate the difference between each value and the sample mean

3. Square the values from step 2
4. Sum the values from step 3
5. Divide by the one less than the sample size

Example 5.4

Suppose the ASC administrator from example 5.1 wishes to use the standard deviation to describe the variation in wait time for patients. Calculate the standard deviation of the 10 wait times 8, 15, 21, 4, 7, 11, 9, 5, 8, 10.

Subject	x_i	$x_i - \bar{x}$	$(x_i - \bar{x})^2$
1	8	(1.80)	3.24
2	15	5.20	27.04
3	21	11.20	125.44
4	4	(5.80)	33.64
5	7	(2.80)	7.84
6	11	1.20	1.44
7	9	(0.80)	0.64
8	5	(4.80)	23.04
9	8	(1.80)	3.24
10	10	0.20	0.04
Sum	98.0	-	225.60
Average	9.8		

$$s^2 = \frac{225.6}{10-1} = 25.1$$

Sample variance = 25.1 minutes^2
Sample standard deviation = 5.0 minutes

Inferential Statistics

Inferential statistics allow generalization from a sample to a population with a certain amount of confidence regarding the findings. Without inferential statistics, it would be very difficult, short of conducting a census, to describe the characteristics of a population.

Note that errors in sampling procedures are inevitable; even with random sampling, there is no guarantee that the sample drawn will be representative of the population. For this reason, inferential statistics are used to allow the variability inherent in the sampling process to be taken into account when making conclusions about a population based on a sample.

As with discrete variables, the primary statistical inference tools used for continuous variables are hypothesis testing and confidence intervals. Hypothesis tests are used to determine if the difference between the observed sample values and the values expected under various hypotheses are different enough so that we are convinced that the difference is more than the amount that may be due to random error. Confidence intervals are a range of values that are likely to include the true population value for a statistic. Both of these tools are used in practice to help analysts make conclusions based on sample data.

One-Sample t-test for the Population Mean

Comparing the mean value of a variable to a standard is common throughout healthcare. A hospital executive may want to understand why the facility's profitability is low for a particular set of services. In order to find the cause of the low profitability, he may request a comparison of the hospital's length of stay to the state average or some other benchmark. Another investigation may require comparing the cost of care for a sample of patients to the payment rate received from an insurance company. Both of these comparisons may be accomplished by using a **one-sample t-test** for the mean.

The steps used in hypothesis testing reviewed in chapter 4 apply here also:

1. Determine the null and alternative hypotheses
2. Set the acceptable type I error or alpha level
3. Select and calculate the appropriate test statistic
4. Compare the test statistic to a critical value based on alpha and the distribution of the test statistic
5. Reject the null hypothesis if the calculated test statistic is more extreme than the critical value. If not, then do not reject the null hypothesis

The null hypothesis is that the population mean is equal to a particular value and the alternative hypothesis is that it is not. This is called a two-sided hypothesis test since the alternative hypothesis is that the population mean is not equal to the null value. If the analyst is only interested in testing to determine if the population mean is less than or greater than a particular value, then a one-sided hypothesis test may be appropriate. The null and alternative hypotheses may be expressed as follows:

For a two-sided hypothesis test: $H_0: \mu = \mu_0$
$H_a: \mu \neq \mu_0$

For a one-sided hypothesis test: $H_0: \mu \leq \mu_0$
$H_a: \mu > \mu_0$

or

$H_0: \mu \geq \mu_0$
$H_a: \mu < \mu_0$

The formula for the one-sample t-test is as follows:

$$t = \frac{\bar{x} - \mu_0}{s/\sqrt{n}}$$

Where $\bar{x}$ is the sample mean, μ_0, is the null hypothesis mean, s is the sample standard deviation and n is the sample size. The critical value for the t-test is determined by the alpha level and degrees of freedom of the test statistic. The degrees of freedom for a one-sample t-test are one less than the sample size, n. Notice that the formulation of the t-test is similar to the hypothesis test statistics presented in chapter 4. The difference between the observed sample value and the null hypothesis value is in the numerator. The denominator is a function of the sample size and the sample standard deviation. The test statistic will take on larger values as the difference between the observed sample value and null hypothesis value increase and as the sample size increases.

The denominator of the t-test is the **standard error of the sample mean**. It is used as a measure of the variation in the data that is scaled for the sample size. Basically, if the sample standard deviation is the same for two samples, the standard error will be smaller for the sample with the larger number of subjects. The standard error is a rough estimate of the precision of the sample mean. In general, larger sample sizes result in a more precise estimate of the population mean and a smaller standard error of the sample mean.

The critical values for the t-test are derived from the t-distribution. The t-distribution is similar to the standard normal distribution in that it is bell-shaped and centered at zero. The t-distribution has a parameter called the degrees of freedom which is similar to that presented for the chi-squared test. In the t-distribution, the degrees of freedom define the width or spread of the bell-shaped curve. As the degrees of freedom increase, the t-distribution curve begins to look like the standard normal. Figure 5.1 shows the t-distribution for various degrees of freedom compared to the standard normal distribution. As the degrees of freedom move from 2 to 5 and finally to 25, the shape of the t-distribution curve moves closer to that of the standard normal distribution.

Figure 5.1 **Comparison of standard normal and t-distribution**

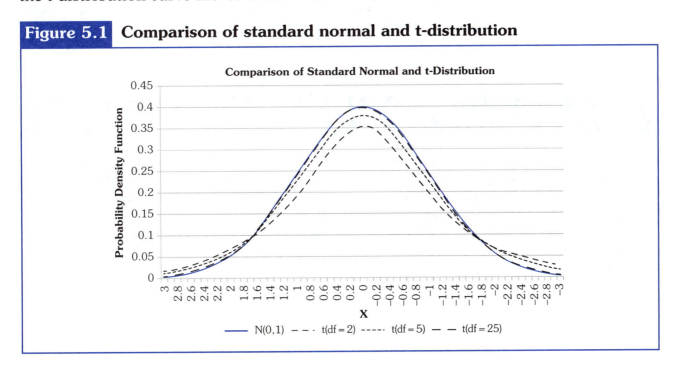

Table 5.1 t-distribution critical values

Degrees of Freedom	Alpha level (use alpha/2 for two sided tests)			
	0.05	0.025	0.01	0.005
1	6.314	12.706	31.821	63.657
2	2.920	4.303	6.965	9.925
3	2.353	3.182	4.541	5.841
4	2.132	2.776	3.747	4.604
5	2.015	2.571	3.365	4.032
6	1.943	2.447	3.143	3.707
7	1.895	2.365	2.998	3.499
8	1.860	2.306	2.896	3.355
9	1.833	2.262	2.821	3.250
10	1.812	2.228	2.764	3.169
15	1.753	2.131	2.602	2.947
20	1.725	2.086	2.528	2.845
25	1.708	2.060	2.485	2.787
30	1.697	2.042	2.457	2.750
35	1.690	2.030	2.438	2.724
50	1.676	2.009	2.403	2.678
100	1.660	1.984	2.364	2.626

Example 5.5 – One-sample t-test for the population mean

A resource utilization consultant wishes to determine if the average length of stay for patients treated for congestive heart failure with major complications and comorbidities (MS-DRG 291) for her client is shorter or longer than the national average of 6.2 days. The consultant selects a sample of 37 patients assigned to MS-DRG 291 and calculates an average length of stay of 4.9 days and a standard deviation of 3.0 days in the sample. Test the hypothesis that the client hospital's length of stay is different from the US average using an alpha level of 0.05.

Example 5.5 – One-sample t-test for the population mean (*continued*)

1. Determine the null and alternative hypotheses

   $H_0: \mu = 6.2$

   $H_a: \mu \neq 6.2$

2. Set the acceptable alpha level: 0.05, two sided test so used 0.05 divided by 2 = 0.025 and $n - 1 = 36$ degrees of freedom to determine critical value

3. Select and calculate the appropriate test statistic

$$t = \frac{\bar{x} - \mu_0}{s/\sqrt{n}} = \frac{4.9 - 6.2}{3.0/\sqrt{37}} = 2.64$$

4. The degrees of freedom for a t-test is $n - 1$ or $37 - 1 = 36$. Table 5.1 lists the critical values for 35 degrees of freedom and alpha divided by 2 = 0.025, 2.030. This serves as an approximation for the critical value for this test. Note that the exact critical value for 36 degrees of freedom and alpha divided by 2 = 0.025 may be found using Excel and the function: = T.INV(0.025,36) which results in the value 2.028.

5. Reject the null hypothesis if the test statistic is greater than 2.030 or less than –2.030. The value of the test statistic is 2.64 which is greater than 2.030. Therefore we reject the null hypothesis and conclude that there is sufficient evidence that the client's length of stay is shorter than the national average at the 0.05 level.

Confidence Interval for the Population Mean

Hypothesis testing is useful to determine if a population is performing different than a standard or benchmark. If an analyst wishes to estimate a reasonable range for the value of a continuous variable, then a confidence interval is the correct statistical tool. The confidence interval is centered at the sample mean and is formulated by adding and subtracting a margin of error based on a critical value and the standard error of the sample mean. The formula for the confidence interval for the population mean with confidence level (1-alpha) is as follows:

$$\bar{x} \pm (critical\ value\ at\ level\ alpha\ /2) \times \frac{s}{\sqrt{n}}$$

Where $\bar{x}$ is the sample mean, s is the sample standard deviation, n is the sample size, and the critical value is from the t-distribution with $n - 1$ degrees of freedom for alphadivided by 2. A 95 percent confidence interval based on a sample size of 6 would require a critical value of 2.571 since alpha = 0.05 and alpha divided by 2 = 0.025.

Example 5.6 – Confidence interval for the population mean

Now that the consultant in example 5.5 knows that the length of stay at her client hospital is less than the national average for MS-DRG 291, she would like to report the value to the hospital's board of directors. Reporting the point estimate or sample mean does inform the board of the precision of the estimate or how sure she is that the estimate is within a particular range. A confidence interval will provide the board with that information. Formulate a 95 percent confidence interval for the mean length of stay for the population of MS-DRG 291 patients at the client hospital. Use the data presented in example 5.5.

Data from example 5.5:

$\bar{x} = 4.9$

$s = 3.0$

$n = 37$

The critical value is the value from table 5.1 where alpha = 0.05 divided by 2 = 0.025 and the degrees of freedom is $n - 1 = 37 - 1 = 36$. We can approximate the critical value from table 5.1 using the value for 35 degrees of freedom, 2.030.

The formula for the confidence interval for the population mean is as follows:

$$\bar{x} \pm (critical\,value\,at\,level\,alpha\,/2) \times \frac{s}{\sqrt{n}}$$

Plugging the values in to the formula:

$$4.9 \pm 2.030 \times \frac{3.0}{\sqrt{37}}$$

$$4.9 \pm 1.0$$

A 95 percent confidence interval for the population mean is 3.9 days to 5.9 days. The consultant may opt to report the interval to the board or report that the mean length of stay is 4.9 days plus or minus one day.

Paired T-test

A **paired t-test** may be used to compare a variable measured at two time points on the same subject. Typically, the measurements are taken before and after an intervention. Some examples include comparing patients' weights before and after a new diet or comparing the length of stay in an intensive care unit (ICU) before and after implementation of a utilization review program. A paired t-test may also be used in comparing values for a variable between matched pairs. Subjects from two population may be matched based on demographics to produce a matched pair to measure the difference in the variable between the two members of the pair. Twins are natural matched pairs.

The null hypothesis in the paired t-test is that there is no difference in the two measurements of the variable. The alternative hypothesis is that there is a difference when comparing the values at the two time points or members of the matched pairs. The null and alternative hypotheses for a paired t-test are expressed as follows :

For a two sided hypothesis test: $H_0: D = d_0$
$H_a: D \neq d_0$

For a one-sided hypothesis test: $H_0: D \leq d_0$
$H_a: D > d_0$
or
$H_0: D \geq d_0$
$H_a: D < d_0$

(Johnson 1997)

The test statistic for the paired t-test is similar to that found in the one-sample t-test. The formula for the test statistic is as follows:

$$t = \frac{\bar{d} - d_0}{s_d / \sqrt{n}}$$

Where $\bar{d}$ is the average of the differences in the sample, s_d is the standard deviation of the differences in the sample, and n is the sample size. Note that 'n' is the number of pairs of values. Notice that this formula is the same as the formula used for the one sample t-test using the differences of the pairs as the variable of interest. The critical value for the test statistic is based on a t-distribution with $n - 1$ degrees of freedom.

Example 5.7 – Paired t-test

The health information management (HIM) Director at Memorial Hospital recently implemented a training program to improve the productivity of their coders. The director selected a sample of six coders and compared the number of outpatient surgery charts coded during an eight-hour shift before and after training. Using the data below, test the hypothesis that the number of charts coded is higher after training than before training at the 0.05 level.

Pre charts	Post charts	d = post charts – pre charts
60	66	6
79	82	3
92	96	4
73	72	-1
75	78	3
80	82	2
69	67	-2

(continued)

Example 5.7 – Paired t-test (*continued*)

1. Determine the null and alternative hypotheses

   $H_0: D \leq 0$

   $H_a: D > 0$

2. Set the acceptable alpha level: 0.05, one-sided test so use alpha = 0.05 and $n - 1 = 6$ degrees of freedom to determine critical value

3. Select and calculate the appropriate test statistic

   (average difference = 2.14; standard deviation difference = 2.79)

   $$t = \frac{\bar{d} - d_0}{s_d / \sqrt{n}} = \frac{2.14 - 0}{2.79 / \sqrt{7}} = 2.03$$

4. From table 5.1, critical value = 1.943

5. Reject the null hypothesis if the test statistic is greater than 1.943. The value of the test statistic is 2.03 which is greater than 1.943. Therefore we reject the null hypothesis and conclude that there is sufficient evidence that the training program improved the number of outpatient surgery charts coded per shift at the 0.05 level.

A confidence interval may be produced to inform the reader of a study of a range of potential values for the difference in the paired values. The formula for the confidence interval of paired differences is as follows:

$$\bar{d} \pm (critical\ value\ at\ level\ alpha\ /2) \times \frac{s_d}{\sqrt{n}}$$

When using confidence interval for paired differences, a one-sided confidence interval may be more appropriate. Often the analyst is only interested in changes in one direction. For instance, in example 5.7, the HIM Director is only interested in how much improvement in productivity is achieved, not how much of a decrease might occur. Therefore, a one-sided confidence interval is more appropriate here. A one-sided lower bound confidence interval is formulated as follows:

$$\bar{d} - (critical\ value\ at\ level\ alpha) \times \frac{s_d}{\sqrt{n}}$$

Notice the two changes to the formula. First, the margin of error is only subtracted from the point estimate and not added and subtracted, since we are only interested in a lower bound. Second, the critical value is now determined by using alpha and not alpha divided by 2. This is because we only are concerned with the confidence on one side of the point estimate.

Example 5.8 – Paired difference confidence interval

The HIM Director in example 5.7 would like to know how much improvement in productivity to expect after the implementation of the training program. She will use the lower bound of the expected improvement for budgeting purposes. Formulate a 95 percent one-sided lower bound confidence interval for the coder productivity data in example 5.6:

$$\bar{d} - (critical\,value\,at\,level\,alpha) \times \frac{s_d}{\sqrt{n}}$$

$$2.10 - 1.943 \times \frac{2.79}{\sqrt{7}}$$

The lower 95 percent confidence bound is $2.14 - 2.05 = 0.9$. The Director may now say she is 95 percent sure that the improvement is at least 0.9 charts per shift. If the HIM department staffs three shifts per day, this results in an improvement of 985 charts over the course of the year.

Two-Sample T-Test

A **two-sample t-test** is a test of a null hypothesis to determine if the means of two groups are statistically different from each other. An analyst may want to compare the lengths of stay in two units of a hospital or two hospitals in the same system. The key difference between the two-sample t-test and the one-sample t-test is that a sample is drawn from two independent populations. The null hypothesis for the two-sample t-test is that the mean of the variable of interest in the two populations is equal. The alternative hypothesis is that they are unequal. The two hypotheses may be expressed in two equivalent ways:

1. The two population means are equal versus not equal:

$H_0: \mu_1 = \mu_2$

$H_a: \mu_1 \neq \mu_2$

2. The difference between the two population means is zero versus not zero:

$H_0: \mu_1 - \mu_2 = 0$

$H_a: \mu_1 - \mu_2 \neq 0$

The second expression is often used because it is an expression that matches the formula for the test statistic required to test the hypothesis. The test statistic for the two-sample t-test follows the same pattern as the test statistics presented previously. The numerator is a measure of difference between the observed sample results and the null hypothesis. The denominator is a measure of the standard error of the point estimate of the population statistic to be tested.

Statistical inference in the field is completed using statistical or spreadsheet software. As the number of populations compared goes beyond one, the formulas become

Example 5.9 – Two-sample t-test

An analyst wanted to find out if the charges for patients admitted through the emergency department (ED) are different from those admitted through other sources. She selected a sample of 12 patients from the population of patients admitted through the ED and those not admitted through the ED. The summary statistics from the samples appear in the table below:

Admitted Through ED?	Sample Average	Sample Standard Deviation	Sample Size
Yes	$ 31,849	$ 8,387	12
No	$ 24,124	$ 8,723	12

Prior to testing the hypothesis using the Excel data analysis toolkit, the analyst performed the five steps to hypothesis testing:

1. Determine the null and alternative hypotheses
   $H_0: \mu_{no} - \mu_{yes} = 0$
   $H_a: \mu_{no} - \mu_{yes} \neq 0$
2. Determine the alpha level: 0.05 (not stated in the example, but a reasonable value)
3. Calculate the test statistic
4. Determine the critical value
   Note: Excel is used for steps 3 and 4. The output appears below:

t-Test: Two-Sample Assuming Equal Variances		
	Not Though ED	*Through ED*
Mean	24,124	31,849
Variance	76,094,440	70,333,470
Observations	12	12
Pooled Variance	73,213,955	
Hypothesized Mean Difference	0	
df	22	
t Stat	(2.211)	
P(T<=t) one-tail	0.019	
t Critical one-tail	1.717	

Example 5.9 – Two-sample t-test (*continued*)

t-Test: Two-Sample Assuming Equal Variances		
	Not Though ED	*Through ED*
P(T<=t) two-tail	0.038	
t Critical two-tail	2.074	

5. Reject the null hypothesis is the test statistic, −2.211, is greater than critical value, 2.074, or less than critical value, −2.074. In this case, −2.211 is less than −2.074. Therefore reject the null hypothesis and conclude that the charges for patients admitted through the ED are significantly higher than those that are not.

increasingly complex. An analyst must understand the five steps to hypothesis testing covered earlier in this chapter even when using statistical software to complete the calculation portion of the analysis. From this point on, this text will concentrate on the interpretation of the output from the Excel data analysis toolkit and statistical package for the social sciences (SPSS) statistical software. A tutorial for using the Excel data analysis toolkit is included in appendix B.

The two-sample t-test may be performed using two sets of assumptions about the population variances for the two populations. Example 5.9 was performed using the assumption that the two population variances are equal. The two sample standard deviations are similar in this case, so the assumption of equal population variances is reasonable here. A formal hypothesis test called **Levene's test** may be used to determine if the variance is different in the two populations. The test statistic used to test the difference between two population means when the variances of the variable in the two populations are unequal does not use the pool variance shown in the Excel output. If we were to rerun the hypothesis test in example 5.9 without assuming equal variances, the conclusion would be the same since the sample variances are so close in value. The results of using the two-sample t-test with unequal variances appear in figure 5.2.

Notice that the output displayed in figure 5.2 does not include the line for pooled variance. Other than that, the test statistic, degrees of freedom, and critical values are all identical.

The SPSS output for the same two-sample t-test is presented in figure 5.3. Notice that the SPSS output also includes the results of Levene's test for the equality of variances. The Excel output does not display this, but instead relies on the user's knowledge of statistics to choose the correct version of the test. The null hypothesis for Levene's test is that the variances of the two populations are equal. In figure 5.3, note that the p-value for that test is 0.715. Recall that we reject a null hypothesis if the p-value is smaller than the alpha level of the hypothesis test. If the alpha level for

Figure 5.2	Excel output for two-sample t-test – assuming unequal variances

t-Test: Two-Sample Assuming Unequal Variances		
	Variable 1	*Variable 2*
Mean	24,124	31,849
Variance	76,094,440	70,333,470
Observations	12	12
Hypothesized Mean Difference	0	
df	22	
t Stat	(2.211)	
P(T<=t) one-tail	0.019	
t Critical one-tail	1.717	
P(T<=t) two-tail	0.038	
t Critical two-tail	2.074	

Levene's test is set to 0.05, then the null hypothesis of equal variances in not rejected. We may then use the top set of results from figure 5.3 and conclude that the hypothesis that the two population means are equal can be rejected at the 0.05 level since the p-value (p = 0.038) is less than 0.05. Notice that the test statistic (t) is –2.211. This is the same value for the test statistic found when using Excel to test the hypothesis of equal population means.

The differences between the t-test for the equality of means with and without assuming equal variances are shown in example 5.10. There are two differences in the statistics displayed for the two versions of the test. First, the degrees of freedom are different for the equal variance assumed and not assumed versions of the test. The smaller degrees of freedom for the version without the assumption of equal variances are part of the adjustment required when the equal variance assumption is not valid. Second, the standard error of the difference between the means is different. This is based on an estimate of the variance of the differences and not the variance pooled across the populations. The different standard error values drive a different test statistic value and finally a different p-value for the two sets of assumptions.

Comparing More Than Two Population Means

The statistical tool used to compare more than two populations is called an **analysis of variance (ANOVA)**. The null hypothesis for an ANOVA is that the population means to be compared are equal. The alternative hypothesis is that at least two of the means

Figure 5.3   SPSS output for two-sample t-test

Independent Samples Test

		Equality of Variance		t-test for Equality of Means						95% Confidence interval of the Difference	
		F	Sig.	t	df	Sig. (2-tailed)	Mean Difference	Std. Error Difference		Lower	Upper
Charge	Equal variances assumed	.136	.715	-2.211	22	.038	(7,724)	3,493		(14,969)	(480)
	Equal variances not assumed			-2.211	21.966	.038	(7,724)	3,493		(14,969)	(479)

are not equal. The hypothesis is tested using an F-statistic. The F-statistic is the ratio of the mean square error between the groups to the mean square error within the groups. If this statistic is large, then the null hypothesis can be rejected. This concept is best demonstrated by examining an example.

All one way ANOVA tables have same structure as demonstrated in example 5.11. The rows in the table represent the type of variance measured: Between Groups, Within Groups, and Total. The sum of the Between Groups Sum of Squares (SS) and the Within Groups SS is equal to the Total SS:

$$17{,}324{,}346{,}245 + 112{,}990{,}114{,}407 = 130{,}314{,}460{,}653$$

The mean square (MS) for each source of variance is equal to the SS divided by the degrees of freedom: $17{,}324{,}346{,}245 \div 2 = 8{,}662{,}173{,}123$ and $112{,}990{,}114{,}407 \div 237 = 476{,}751{,}538$. Finally, the test statistic, F, is equal to the MS Between divided by MS Within: $8{,}662{,}173{,}123 \div 476{,}751{,}538 = 18.17$. The p-value is then derived by comparing the value of the F-statistic to the F-distribution with 2 and 237 degrees of freedom. A generalization of the one-way ANOVA table appears in figure 5.4.

The conclusion of the ANOVA in example 5.11 is to reject the null hypothesis and conclude that at least two of the population means are different. The next natural question is: "Which means are different?" That question can be answered by performing

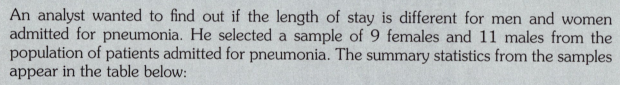

Example 5.10 – Two-sample t-test – unequal variances

An analyst wanted to find out if the length of stay is different for men and women admitted for pneumonia. He selected a sample of 9 females and 11 males from the population of patients admitted for pneumonia. The summary statistics from the samples appear in the table below:

Gender	N	Sample Mean	Standard Deviation
M	11	7.18	4.73
F	9	3.33	2.12

Prior to testing the hypothesis using Excel, the analyst performed the five steps to hypothesis testing:

1. Determine the null and alternative hypotheses
   $H_0: \mu_{female} - \mu_{male} = 0$
   $H_a: \mu_{female} - \mu_{male} \neq 0$
2. Determine the alpha level: 0.05 (not stated in the example, but a reasonable value)
3. Calculate the test statistic
4. Determine the critical value
   Note: SPSS is used for steps 3 and 4. The output appears below:

Example 5.10 – Two-sample t-test – unequal variances (continued)

Independent Samples Test

		Levene's Test for Equality of Variance		t-test for Equality of Means					Confidence	
		F	Sig.	t	df	Sig. (2-tailed)	Mean Difference	Std. Error Difference	Lower	Upper
LOS	Equal variances assumed	5.033	.038	2.25	18.00	.037	3.85	1.71	0.26	7.43
	Equal variances not assumed			2.42	14.43	.029	3.85	1.59	0.44	7.25

In this case, the p-value for Levene's test is 0.038. The hypothesis for the equality of the means is rejected, so we must use the test results on the line titled "equal variances not assumed." Reject the null hypothesis that the two population means are equal since the p-value for the t-test for equality of means, 0.029, is smaller than the pre-set alpha level of 0.05.

Figure 5.4   ANOVA example

Source of Variation	SS	df	MS	F
Between Groups	SSb	DFb	MSB = SSB/DFb	MSB/MSW
Within Groups	SSw	DFw	MSW = SSW/DFw	
Total	SSt	DFt		

Example 5.11 – Analysis of variance

The Medicare severity-adjusted diagnosis-related group (MS-DRG) system is designed so that the level of resources as measured by charges per patient required to treat a patient are different within the no complication or comorbidity (CC) or major complication or comorbidity (MCC) family. An analyst was asked to test to see if that relationship was true at her facility. A sample of 80 cases was selected for the three congestive heart failure MS-DRGs: 291 (MCC), 292 (CC), 293 (no CC or MCC). Since three populations of patients are compared, the analyst used Excel to generate summary statistics and the ANOVA table below.

Anova: Single Factor

SUMMARY

Groups	Count	Sum	Average	Variance
291	80	3,550,238	44,378	733,847,198
292	80	2,609,870	32,623	572,536,931
293	80	1,890,221	23,628	123,870,483

ANOVA

Source of Variation	SS	df	MS	F	P-value
Between Groups	17,324,346,245	2	8,662,173,123	18.17	0.000
Within Groups	112,990,114,407	237	476,751,538		
Total	130,314,460,653	239			

Notice that the sample averages all appear to be quite different. The variances are also different. An ANOVA includes an assumption that the variance in the populations are equal, but ANOVA is considered to be valid in the face of unequal variances if the

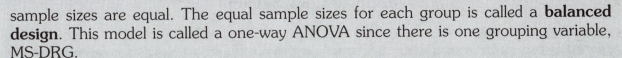

Example 5.11 – Analysis of variance (continued)

sample sizes are equal. The equal sample sizes for each group is called a **balanced design**. This model is called a one-way ANOVA since there is one grouping variable, MS-DRG.

Use five steps of hypothesis testing:

1. The null hypothesis and alternative hypotheses are

   H_0: $\mu_{291} = \mu_{292} = \mu_{293}$

   H_a: at least two means are not equal

2. Set the significance level: 0.05
3. Calculate the test statistic: $F = 18.17$ from ANOVA table
4. Determine the critical value. Excel reports the p-value as < 0.0001. Note: a p-value is never reported as zero.
5. Reject the null hypothesis and conclude that at least two of the MS-DRG average charges are different at the 0.05 level since the p-value is < 0.05.

a post hoc analysis. A **Tukey Honest Significant Difference (HSD) test** is the most common type of post hoc analysis used in practice. Excel does not have the capacity to perform a Tukey analysis as part of the analysis toolpak, but SPSS has the capability to perform the test.

The ANOVA output in figure 5.5 includes an ANOVA table and the output of the Tukey HSDTest. The values in the ANOVA table match those presented in example 5.11 from Excel. The Tukey HSD post hoc test allows us to determine which MS-DRGs are likely to have different average charges. The Tukey HSD output presents the pairwise

Figure 5.5 SPSS ANOVA output

ANOVA

Charge

	Sum of Squares	df	Mean Square	F	Sig.
Between Groups	17,324,346,245	2	8,662,173,123	18,169	.000
Within Groups	112,990,114,407	237	476,751,538		
Total	130,314,460,653	239			

(continued)

Figure 5.5	SPSS ANOVA output (*continued*)

Multiple Comparisons

Charge Tukey HSD

(I) MSDRG	(J) MSDRG	Mean Difference (I-J)	Std. Error	Sig.	95% Confidence Interval Lower Bound	Upper Bound
291	292	11,755	3,452	0.002	3,612	19,897
	293	20,750	3,452	0.000	12,608	28,893
292	291	(11,755)	3,452	0.002	(19,897)	(3,612)
	293	8,996	3,452	0.026	853	17,138
293	291	(20,750)	3,452	0.000	(28,893)	(12,608)
	292	(8,996)	3,452	0.026	(17,138)	(853)

differences for all of the means, the p-value for the hypothesis test that the two means are different and finally a 95 percent confidence interval for the difference between the pair of means. The first row compares the average charge for MS-DRGs 291 and 292. The hypothesis that the 291 and 292 means are equal is rejected since the p-value, 0.002, is smaller than the preset alpha level of 0.05. Similarly, the average charge for 291 and 293 are different with a p-value < 0.001. Finally, the comparison of 292 and 293 is presented on the fourth row of the table. Since the p-value for all three of the pairwise comparisons are below 0.05, we can conclude that all the population means for all three populations are different at the 0.05 level.

✔ Review Questions

1. Which of the following measures of central tendency is least influenced by outliers?
   a. Mean
   b. Median
   c. Mode
   d. Quartile

2. Which of these statistics is a measure of spread?
   a. Mean
   b. Median
   c. Minimum
   d. Standard deviation

3. Which statistical tool should be used to determine if there is a significant difference in the lengths of stay for three hospitals?

   a. Confidence interval
   b. Levene's test
   c. Analysis of Variance
   d. Two sample t-test

4. What is the median of the following numbers: 3, 9, 2, 5, 5

   a. 3
   b. 9
   c. 1
   d. 5

5. What is the mean of the following numbers: 3, 9, 2, 5, 5

   a. 9
   b. 5.5
   c. 4.8
   d. 2.5

6. What is the range of the following numbers: 3, 9, 2, 5, 5

   a. 5
   b. 7
   c. 9
   d. 2

7. An analyst wishes to test the hypothesis that the wait time in the Department is longer on weekends than week days. What is the alternative hypothesis?

   a. Average wait time is shorter on weekends
   b. Average wait time is longer on weekends
   c. Average wait time is different on weekends and weekdays
   d. Average wait time is the same on weekends and weekdays.

8. An analyst calculates a t-test statistic for testing the null hypothesis that the wait time in the Emergency Department is longer on weekends than week days. The test statistic is based on a sample of 50 patients from each population and is equal to 3.92. If the alpha level is set to 0.01, should the null hypothesis be rejected?

   a. Yes
   b. No
   c. Not enough information

9. The standard normal distribution and the t-distribution are both:

   a. Bell shaped
   b. Symmetric
   c. Centered at zero
   d. All of the above

10. An analyst wishes to test the impact of a new patient schedule system on number of MRI tests performed per day. What statistical test should be used?
    a. T-test
    b. Two-sample t-test
    c. ANOVA
    d. Paired t-test

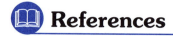 # References

Johnson, W. 1997. *Business Statistics: Decision Making with Data*. New York: John Wiley & Sons.

Analyzing the Relationship between Two Variables

KEY TERMS

Coefficient of determination	Simple linear regression
Correlation	Slope intercept form
Least squares regression line	Spearman's Rho
Pearson's r Correlation Coefficient	Standardized residuals
Residual	T-test for correlations
R-square	

Correlation

A data analyst may be asked to assess the relationship between two variables. **Correlation** is the statistic that is used to describe the association or relationship between two continuous variables. In the healthcare setting, we may note that length of stay and charges are closely related or correlated. Since charges increase as length of stay increases, we say that the two variables are positively correlated. An example of two variables that are negatively correlated may be years of coder experience and time to code a health record. If the more experienced coders have shorter review times, then the two variables are negatively correlated.

It is important to note that correlation and causation are two very different concepts. Causation is far more difficult to prove via data and really requires a carefully designed and controlled experiment to prove. Correlation or association between two variables may be identified in both observational and designed studies.

Descriptive Statistics

Pearson's r Correlation Coefficient

Pearson's r Correlation Coefficient (r) measures the strength of the linear relationship between two continuous variables. The statistic can range from -1 to $+1$. Negative one is a perfect negative correlation while positive one is a perfect positive correlation. The formula for calculating the statistic is:

$$r = \frac{\sum_{i=1}^{n}(X_i - \bar{X})(Y_i - \bar{Y})}{\sqrt{\sum_{i=1}^{n}(X_i - \bar{X})^2}\sqrt{\sum_{i=1}^{n}(Y_i - \bar{Y})^2}}.$$

(Johnson 1997)

Notice that the numerator of the statistic will determine the sign of the correlation. Confidence intervals and hypothesis tests may be performed to make inference about the strength of association between two variables.

Example 6.1 – Pearson's correlation coefficient

As coders gain more experience, they should be able to code records more quickly. In order to quantify that relationship, an analyst selected a sample of seven coders. For the subjects sampled, the years of experience and average time to code an outpatient records was collected. The data from the study appear in the table below:

Subject	Experience (years)	Time (minutes)
1	5	30
2	1	60
3	2	45
4	5	35
5	3	45
6	2	39
7	3	37

Experience will be labeled as X and time to code will be labeled Y. The first step in calculating the Pearson Correlation Coefficient is to calculate the average years of experience and time to code:

$$\bar{X} = \frac{5+1+2+5+3+2+3}{7} = \frac{21}{7} = 3.0$$

$$\bar{Y} = \frac{30+60+45+35+45+39+37}{7} = \frac{291}{7} = 41.6$$

The calculation of r is easiest to complete using a table format:

Subject	X:Experience (years)	Y:Time (minutes)	$X-\bar{X}$	$\bar{Y}$	$(X-\bar{X})^2$	$(Y-\bar{Y})^2$	$(X-\bar{X}) \times (Y-\bar{Y})$
1	5	30	2.0	(11.6)	4.0	133.9	(23.1)
2	1	60	(2.0)	18.4	4.0	339.6	(36.9)
3	2	45	(1.0)	3.4	1.0	11.8	(3.4)
4	5	35	2.0	(6.6)	4.0	43.2	(13.1)
5	3	45	0.0	3.4	0.0	11.8	-
6	2	39	(1.0)	(2.6)	1.0	6.6	2.6
7	3	37	0.0	(4.6)	0.0	20.9	-
Sum	21	291	0.0	0.0	14.0	567.7	(74.0)
Average	3.0	41.6					

$$r = \frac{-74.0}{\sqrt{14.0} \times \sqrt{567.7}} = -0.83$$

The value of Pearson's correlation coefficient, −0.83, is indicative of a negative relationship between experience and time to code a record. In other words, the negative sign on r means that as experience increases, the time to code a record decreases. A value of negative one would mean there was a perfect inverse linear relationship between the two variables. A value of −0.83 represents a very strong negative correlation. The relationship is displayed as a scatter plot in figure 6.1.

Figure 6.1   Pearson's correlation coefficient

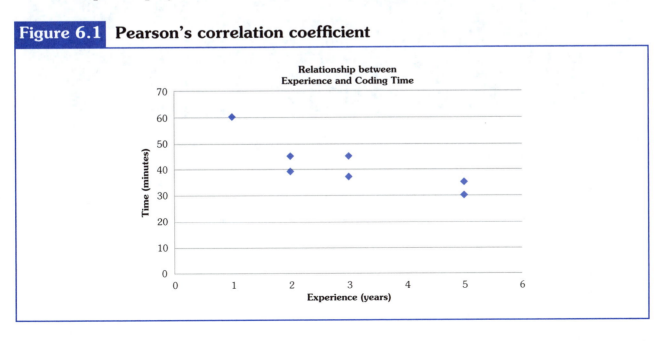

Spearman's Rho Correlation Coefficient

Pearson's r correlation coefficient is appropriate to use when describing the linear relationship between two interval or ratio variables. It is not appropriate to use Pearson's r when one or both of the variables are ordinal. Recall that ordinal variables are categorical, but have a natural order. Healthcare data includes a number of examples of ordinal variables such as: patient severity, trauma levels and patient satisfaction scores collected on a Likert scale. **Spearman's Rho** is calculated based on the relative ranks of the two variables. The range for Spearman's Rho is from −1 to 1 and is interpreted the same as Pearson's r. The formula for Spearman's Rho is the same as the formula for Pearson's r, but the X and Y values represent the ranks of each series of data. If there are no ties in the ranking of the variables, then the following formula may be used (Osborn 2006):

$$r_{rho} = 1 - \frac{6 \times \sum_i D_i}{n \times (n^2 - 1)}$$

Where D_i is the difference between the ranks of the ith pair of variables and n is the sample size.

Example 6.2 – Spearman's Rho

Hospitals bill for emergency department (ED) visits based on current procedural terminology (CPT) codes for levels 1 through 5. A hospital's ED Director would like to verify that the methodology used for assigning levels to patients is positively correlated with the resources required to treat the patient. The resources are measured by the total charge for the ED visit for items associated with the ED services. The director selected a sample of seven patients and recorded the level assigned to the ED visit (one to five) and the ED service charges. The data is presented in the table below:

ED Level (X)	Charge (Y)	Rank X	Rank Y	Rank X – Average Rank X	Rank Y – Average Rank Y	Rank X – Average Rank X squared	Rank Y – Average Rank Y squared	(Rank X – Average Rank X) × (Rank Y – Average Rank Y)
1	1500	1	1	−3	−3	9	9	9
4	2709	5.5	5	1.5	1	2.25	1	1.5
5	3251	7	7	3	3	9	9	9

ED Level (X)	Charge (Y)	Rank X	Rank Y	Rank X – Average Rank X	Rank Y – Average Rank Y	Rank X – Average Rank X squared	Rank Y – Average Rank Y squared	(Rank X – Average Rank X) × (Rank Y – Average Rank Y)
4	2106	5.5	2	1.5	-2	2.25	4	-3
2	2585	2.5	4	-1.5	0	2.25	0	0
2	2513	2.5	3	-1.5	-1	2.25	1	1.5
3	3210	4	6	0	2	0	4	0
Totals		28	28	0	0	27	28	18
Average		4	4					

Since the ED levels are ordinal, a Spearman's Rho statistic should be used to measure the correlation between the two variables. Notice that there are a number of ties in the ranking of the ED levels. Therefore, the calculation of Spearman's Rho is performed using the formula for Pearson's r using the ranks for the two variables:

$$r_{rho} = \frac{18}{\sqrt{27} \times \sqrt{28}} = 0.65$$

There is a positive correlation between the ED level and resources used in the ED.

Inferential Statistics

Correlations close to one or negative one indicate strong positive or negative correlations. A **t-test for correlations** may be performed to test the null hypothesis that the correlation between two variables is zero. The hypothesis test formula is the same for Pearson's r and Spearman's Rho. The formula is:

$$t = r \times \frac{\sqrt{(n-2)}}{\sqrt{1-r^2}}$$

where r is either the value of Pearson's r or Spearman's Rho and n is the sample size. The test statistic, t, should be compared to the t-distribution with $n - 2$ degrees of freedom.

Notice that the sample size is in the numerator of the test statistic for testing the statistical significance of a correlation. The value of the test statistic is proportional to

Example 6.3 – Testing hypothesis that Pearson's r is zero

Test the hypothesis that the correlation between coder experience and minutes to code a record is zero at the 0.05 level.

1. State the null and alternative hypothesis

   H_0: r = 0

   H_a: r ≠ 0

2. Set the acceptable alpha level: 0.05, two sided test so used 0.05 ÷ 2 = 0.025 and n − 2 = 5 degrees of freedom to determine critical value from table 5.1.

3. Select and calculate the appropriate test statistic

$$t = r \times \frac{\sqrt{(n-2)}}{\sqrt{1-r^2}} = -0.83 \times \frac{\sqrt{(7-2)}}{\sqrt{1-(-0.83)^2}} = -3.33$$

4. Compare −3.33 to critical value from table 5.1: 2.447. Reject the null hypothesis if the test statistic is greater than 2.447 or less than −2.447.

5. The value of the test statistic is −3.33 which is less than −2.447. Therefore we reject the null hypothesis and conclude that there is sufficient evidence that the correlation is significantly different from zero at the 0.05 level.

Example 6.4 – Testing hypothesis that Spearman's Rho is zero

Test the hypothesis that the correlation between ED Level and resource intensity is zero at the 0.05 level.

1. State the null and alternative hypothesis

   H_0: rho = 0

   H_a: rho ≠ 0

2. Set the acceptable alpha level: 0.05, two sided test so used 0.05 ÷ 2 = 0.025 and n − 2 = 5 degrees of freedom to determine critical value from table 5.1.

3. Select and calculate the appropriate test statistic

$$t = rho \times \frac{\sqrt{(n-2)}}{\sqrt{1-rho^2}} = 0.65 \times \frac{\sqrt{(7-2)}}{\sqrt{1-(0.65)^2}} = 1.10$$

4. Compare 1.10 to critical value from table 5.1: 2.447. Reject the null hypothesis if the test statistic is greater than 2.447 or less than −2.447.

5. The value of the test statistic is 1.10 which is not greater than 2.447. Therefore we do not reject the null hypothesis and conclude that there is not sufficient evidence that the correlation is significantly different from zero at the 0.05 level.

the square root of the sample size minus 2. This means that the correlation of 0.65 may have been considered significantly different from zero with a larger sample size. For this reason, the statistical significance of the T-test for correlations may not identify practical significance in the relationship between two variables when the sample size is very large.

Simple Linear Regression

When examining the correlation between two variables, the strength and direction of the relationship is measured. The next step in exploring the relationship between two variables is to analyze the ability of the value of one variable to predict an outcome or value of a second variable. In this scenario, the variable that is used to predict is called the independent variable. The outcome or variable to be predicted is called the dependent variable. An easy way to recall which variable is dependent or independent is to remember that the dependent variable *depends* on the value of the independent variable. For instance, inpatient length of stay and total charges for an inpatient stay are positively correlated for most types of admissions, but is length of stay a good predictor of total charge? In this scenario, length of stay is the independent variable and total charge is the dependent variable. Note that even if an independent variable is an excellent predictor of a dependent variable, that relationship does not necessarily mean that there is a cause and effect relationship.

Simple linear regression is used to characterize the linear relationship between a dependent variable and one independent variable. The regression line is typically expressed in a **slope intercept form**:

$$Y = BX + A$$

In this formula, B represents the slope of the line and A represents the y-intercept. The slope of a line represents the amount of change in the dependent variable, Y, for every one unit change in the independent variable, x. The y-intercept represents the point where the line intercepts the y-axis or the value of the dependent variable when the independent variable is equal to zero.

In figure 6.2, the line that represents the relationship between coder experience and time to code a record is represented by the line: $Y = -5.29 \times X + 57.43$ or time = -5.29 x experience + 57.43. Notice that the slope of the line is negative. The Pearson's r for these two variables was calculated to be -0.83 in example 6.1. The sign of the slope of the regression line is always the same as the sign on the correlation coefficient of the two variables. The slope of the regression line, -5.29, may be interpreted as the change in time to code records corresponding to the change in the number of years of experience. According to the regression line fit to the data, a coder's time should be reduced by 5.29 minutes for every year of experience. The y-intercept of the regression line, 57.43 may be interpreted as the time to code records for a coder with no years of experience.

The regression line depicted in figure 6.2 is called a **least squares regression line**. An in depth study of the formula used to determine the least squares regression line is beyond the scope of this text, but it is useful to understand the intuition behind the

Figure 6.2 **Regression line example**

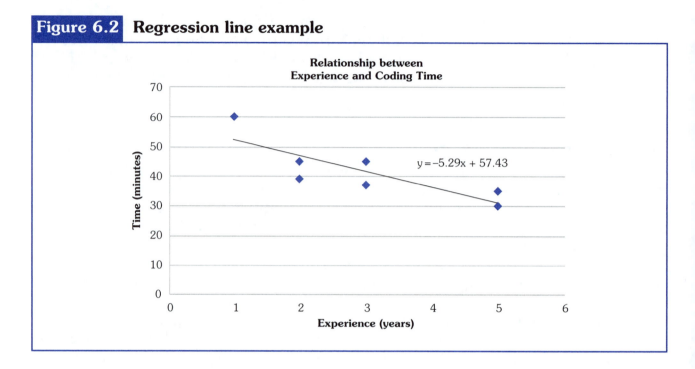

fitting of the least squares or best fit regression line. Notice that the line does not actually go through any of the seven data points, but it does come very close to all of them. The vertical distance between the regression line and each data point is called the regression error. There are two coders with three years of experience. Using the regression line, we can predict the value of their coding time: $y = -5.29 \times 3 + 57.43 = 41.56$. Referring back to example 6.1, the time values for the two coders with three years of experience are 37 and 45 minutes. The regression line did not exactly predict the values, but came close to both values.

A representation of the least squares regression line is:

$$Y = bX + a + e$$

Where b is the slope and a is the intercept, estimate from the least squares regression line and e is the error term or **residual**. Figure 6.3 is a rescaled version of figure 6.2. The dashed vertical lines represent the error term resulting from the least squares regression line. The least squares line is the line that minimizes the sum of the squared error values. The line should be as close as possible to all points and not above or below all of them, so the value to be minimized is the squared error values to remove the positive or negative sign from the residual. The line depicted in figures 6.2 and 6.3 minimizes the sum of the squared errors or vertical distance between the line and all of the points.

Before using a least squares regression line to predict values of a dependent variable, there are a number of assumptions about the error term that must be checked. The most important assumption to check in simple linear regression is that the error terms are approximately normally distributed around zero. Recall that the normal distribution is the formal name for a bell shaped curve. If the error terms are normally distributed around zero, then there must be some positive and negative error values and most of the values are grouped near the average of zero.

Figure 6.3   Least squares error demonstration

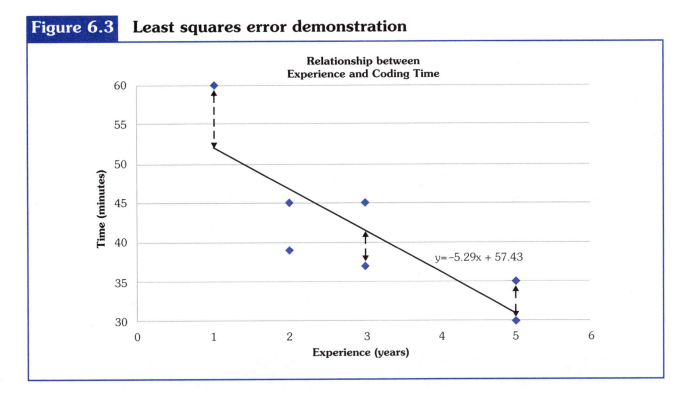

Satisfying this assumption ensures that the regression line is not biased by extreme values. In the coder experience versus time to code regression, the violation of this assumption may mean that the time to code is over estimated for more values of experience than it is underestimated. This assumption can be checked graphically by generating a histogram of the standardized residuals or by performing a formal test of normality. **Standardized residuals** are created by subtracting the average residual and dividing by the standard deviation of the residuals. Most statistical analysis software tools include the ability to check this and other assumptions required for simple linear regression.

The regression statistics portion of the Excel summary output includes two important statistics: multiple R and R-square. Multiple R in the case of simple linear regression is the Pearson's correlation coefficient between the dependent and independent variable. The **R-square** is sometimes referred to as the coefficient of determination. The **coefficient of determination** measures the amount of variance in the dependent variable that is explained by the independent variable. In example 6.5, the correlation between length of stay and total charge is 0.78. Length of stay explains 61 percent of the variance in charges (0.78^2). This means that other factors explain the remaining 39 percent of the variance in charges, but 61 percent is explained by length of stay alone.

The ANOVA portion of the Excel output presents the results of testing the null hypothesis that the slope of the line is zero versus the slope of the line is not zero. In a regression with one independent variable, this is equivalent to the hypothesis test listed in the coefficient portion of the output. The coefficient portion of the output tests two null hypotheses: Is the intercept of the regression line equal to zero?; Is the slope of the line equal to zero? These are important hypotheses to test. If the y-intercept is equal to zero, then that term does not need to be included in the line. If the slope of the regression line is not significantly different from zero, then the independent variable is not helpful in predicting the dependent variable and that term should not be included in the model.

If we set our acceptable alpha level to be 0.05 in example 6.5, then the null hypothesis that the y-intercept is zero may be rejected at the p-value 0.0072. The null hypothesis that the slope is zero may also be rejected at the alpha equal 0.05 level (p-value < 0.0001). The results of these two hypotheses tests and the lack of any evidence that the

Example 6.5 – Simple linear regression – Excel output

A healthcare data analyst working for a commercial payer requested historical length of stays and charge data for a sample of patients admitted to a local hospital. The goal was to predict the total charge for a patient based on the length of stay using simple linear regression. The sample included data for 37 patients. The analyst used the Excel data analysis toolkit to fit the least squares regression line. The output appears below:

SUMMARY OUTPUT

Regression Statistics	
Multiple R	0.78
R Square	0.61
Adjusted R Square	0.59
Standard Error	10,611
Observations	37

ANOVA

	df	SS	MS	F	Significance F
Regression	1	6,066,384,346	6,066,384,346	53.87	< 0.0001
Residual	35	3,941,118,051	112,603,373		
Total	36	10,007,502,397			

	Coefficients	Standard Error	t Start	P-value	Lower 95%	Upper 95%
Intercept	9,582	3,357.03	2.85	0.0072	2,767	16,397
LOS	4,303	586.31	7.34	< 0.0001	3,113	5,494

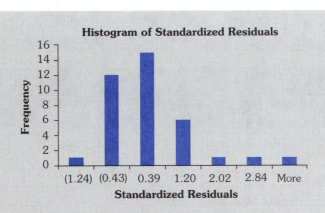

The shaded box in the Summary Output from the Excel Data Analysis Toolkit shows displays the coefficients for the least squared regression line: Charge = 4303x LOS + 9582. The LOS Residual Plot and Histogram of Standardized Residuals show that the errors are approximately normally distributed and meet the assumptions for least squares regression. The Summary Output contains much more information that is explained below.

residuals are non normal lead to the conclusion that the regression line will result in a useful estimate for total charges based on length of stay.

The output from **SPSS** results in the same values as that found in the Excel output. SPSS has the functionality to perform the residual histogram built in while a separate step was required to produce that graph in Excel. As models become more complex and include multiple independent variables, statistical software should be used to perform the analysis. Excel is capable of producing a multiple regression equation, but it is not well suited for testing many of the assumptions that are required when modeling beyond simple linear regression.

Example 6.6 – Simple linear regression – SPSS output

The analyst repeated the fit of the least squares regression line using Statistical Package for the Social Sciences (SPSS). The output appears below:

Model Summary				
Model	R	R Square	Adjusted R Square	Std. Error of the Estimate
1	.779	.606	.595	10,611.47

(continued)

Example 6.6 – Simple linear regression – SPSS output (*continued*)

ANOVA

Model		Sum of Squares	df	Mean Square	F	Sig.
1	Regression	6,066,384,346	1	6,066,384,346	53.874	.000
	Residual	3,941,118,051	35	112,603,373		
	Total	10,007,502,397	36			

Coefficients

Model		Unstandardized Coefficients		Stand-ard-ized Coeffi-cients			95.0% Confi-dence Interval for B	
		B	Std. Error	Beta	t	Sig.	Lower Bound	Upper Bound
1	(Constant)	9,582	3,357		2.854	.007	2,767	16,397
	LOS	4,303	586	.779	7.340	.000	3,113	5,494

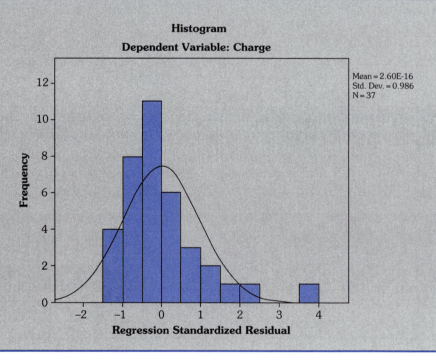

Histogram

Dependent Variable: Charge

Mean = 2.60E-16
Std. Dev. = 0.986
N = 37

Review Questions

1. The statistic that measures association between two interval type variables is:
   a. Chi-squared
   b. Pearson's r
   c. Proportion
   d. Spearman's Rho

2. If length of stay and charges are positively correlated, then which of the following is true:
   a. As length of stay increases charges decrease
   b. As length of stay increases charges increase
   c. Length of stay and charges are not related
   d. As length of stay increases charges do not change

3. The statistic that is used to measure association between an ordinal and an interval variable is:
   a. Chi-squared
   b. Pearson's r
   c. Proportion
   d. Spearman's Rho

4. In the slope intercept form of a regression line: $Y = BX + A$, what is the interpretation of the slope?
   a. The point that the line intersects with the y-axis
   b. The change in Y for every one unit change in X
   c. The point that the line intersects with the x-axis
   d. The change in X for every one unit change in Y

5. Linear regression was used to estimate the relationship between the number of laboratory tests performed on a patient during a stay (Y) and the number of days spent in the ICU (X). The estimated regression equation was: $Y = 10 + 6 \times X$. Estimate the number of laboratory tests expected for a patient that spent 3 days in the ICU.
   a. 6
   b. 10
   c. 28
   d. 18

6. If the correlation between X and Y is 0.90, what is the correlation between Y and X?
   a.   0.90
   b. −0.90
   c.   0.10
   d. −0.10

7. If the correlation between two variables is virtually the same when drawing a sample of $n = 10$ as it is when a sample of size $n = 100$ is drawn, what impact does the larger sample size have on the T-test for testing the null hypothesis that a population correlation is zero?

   a. The test statistic increases
   b. The test statistic stays the same
   c. The test statistic decreases
   d. Not enough information given

8. The correlation between time to code a health record and the dates of service is 0.76. If a regression line is fit using time to code as the dependent variable and dates of service as the independent variable, what is the coefficient of determination?

   a. 0.76
   b. 0.38
   c. 0.87
   d. 0.58

9. What are the assumptions regarding the residuals in simple linear regression?

   a. Residuals have a mean of zero
   b. Residuals are approximately normally distributed
   c. Standardized residuals follow the standard normal distribution
   d. All of the above

10. Least squares estimate the regression line by:

   a. Selecting a line that crosses all points
   b. Minimizing the squared distance from the points to the line
   c. Minimizing the total distance from points to the line
   d. Selecting a line that connects the minimum and maximum Y values

📖 References

Johnson, W. 1997. *Business Statistics: Decision Making with Data*. New York: John Wiley & Sons.

Osborn, C.E. 2006. *Statistical Applications for Health Information Management*, 2nd ed. Sudbury: Jones and Bartlett Publishers.

Sample Selections

KEY TERMS

Cluster random sampling	Sample
Convenience sampling	Sampling frame
Judgment sampling	Sampling plan
Non probability sampling	Simple random sampling
Population	Strata
Probability sampling	Stratified random sampling
Quota sampling	Systematic random sample
Random seed	Universe

Vocabulary of Sampling

The analysis techniques described in this text thus far relied on the collection of a simple random sample from a larger population. Descriptive statistics may be used to describe the sample and inferential statistics may be used to generalize the results found in the sample to the larger population. Sampling is used when examining the entire population is either too time consuming or too expensive. In many scenarios, an analyst may not have access to the entire population either because services are ongoing and continuously adding to the population or there is no listing of the population available.

A **sample** is the subset of a **population** or universe. The **universe** is the set of all units that are eligible to be sampled. A listing of all of the subjects in the universe is called the **sampling frame**. The universe in a sampling plan may be patients, physicians, health records, or any other unit of analysis that is studied. A **sampling plan** includes a definition of the population, any inclusion or exclusion criteria, and the sampling methodology. The variable of interest or quantity to be estimated should be determined prior to developing a sampling plan. If the goal of a study is to estimate a coding error rate, then the unit of analysis may be the codes assigned to an account. If the goal is to estimate the rate of Medicare serverity-adjusted diagnosis-related group (MS-DRG) changes due to a detailed record review, then the unit of analysis is the account or claim. The variable of interest should be defined carefully because it will drive the unit of analysis and the universe to be sampled.

Sample selections are made based on one of two sampling methods. "In **probability sampling**, each member of a population has a known probability of being selected for the sample. **Non-probability sampling** is that in which members of a sample are deliberately selected for a specified purpose" (Osborn 2006, 139). If the goal of the analysis is to gain an understanding of a process or exploratory data analysis, then a non probability sample may be used. The goal of the study should be determined prior to the collection of any data. If the goal is to generalize the results from the sample to the population then a probability sample should be used.

Sample Selection Techniques

Probability sampling includes simple random sampling, stratified random sampling, systematic sampling, and cluster sampling. Non probability sampling includes quota sampling, convenience sampling, and judgment sampling. If the goal of the analysis is to generalize the results of the analysis of the sample to the full population, then a probability sample is appropriate.

The term "statistically valid sample" is used often in practice. In order for a sample to be statistically valid, it must be large enough to provide information with sufficient precision to meet the goals of the analysis. Guidelines for selecting a sample size are discussed later in this chapter. A statistically valid sample is typically a probability sample where each item in the population has an equal chance of being selected. Finally, a

---

Example 7.1 – Defining the variable of interest

A director of a physician practice suspects that the physicians may not be signing the orders for magnetic resonance imagings (MRIs) performed on site. The practice only performs MRIs on patients treated by their staff physicians. She wishes to generalize her conclusions to determine the proportion of MRI tests ordered by physicians at the practice that were not signed over the last year. Define the variable of interest, population, and appropriate type of sampling to be performed.

The variable of interest is the proportion of MRI orders unsigned. The proportion is defined by a denominator and numerator:

>   Numerator: Number of unsigned MRIs ordered by physicians at the practice and performed on site over the last year.

>   Denominator: Total number of MRIs performed on site over the last year.

The population is all MRIs performed on site over the last year. The denominator of the proportion defines the population for the sampling plan.

The director should use a probability sample so that she may generalize the results to the full population.

statistically valid sample is reproducible. A reader or end user should be able to recreate the sample with the documentation provided by the analyst who selected the sample.

Centers for Medicare and Medicaid Services (CMS) defines the following documentation should be maintained when generating a sample for the purposes of performing an audit:

> 3.10.4.4.1 - Documentation of Universe and Frame
>
> (Rev. 282, Issued: 01-08-09, Effective: 01-26-09, Implementation: 01-26-09)
>
> An explicit statement of how the universe is defined and elements included shall be made and maintained in writing. Further, the form of the frame and specific details as to the period covered, definition of the sampling unit(s), identifiers for the sampling units (e.g., claim numbers, carrier control numbers), and dates of service and source shall be specified and recorded in your record of how the sampling was done. A record shall be kept of the random numbers actually used in the sample and how they were selected. Sufficient documentation shall be kept so that the sampling frame can be re-created, should the methodology be challenged.
>
> (CMS 2011).

The attributes of the documentation of the universe and sampling provided by CMS are an excellent guideline for best practices.

Probability Sampling Techniques

Simple Random Sampling

In **simple random sampling**, every member of the population has an equal chance of being selected for the sample. Simple random sampling is the statistical equivalent of drawing sampling units from a hat. The sample can be chosen through a random drawing or by numbering the population and making choices through the use of random number tables or a random number generator. If a random number generator is used, then a seed should be set so that the sample can be replicated. Every random number generator has a starting point, or **random seed.** If the seed is designated and recorded as part of the sampling plan, then the series of random numbers can be replicated by another analyst using the same software and seed. The steps in selecting a simple random sample are:

1. Assign a sequential number as a row label to every unit in the sampling frame.
2. Select a series of random integers between 1 and n, where n is the sample size.

or

1. Assign a random number to each unit in the sampling frame.
2. Order the units by the random number.
3. Select the first n as the sample, where n is the sample size.

The second strategy works well in Excel. When using Excel to generate random numbers, do not use the RAND() function. The RAND() function does not allow the user to assign a seed to generate the random numbers. The system time from the computer used to generate the sample is used as the seed for RAND(). Therefore two samples must be created at exactly the same time on two computer that have their system times synced in order to reproduce the sample. Instead use the "Random Number Generation" feature in the Data Analysis Toolpak. Random numbers are generated base on a probability distribution. All of the distributions available in the Excel Random Number generation feature allow the selection of a random seed except discrete and pattern. Those two choices should not be used when creating a sample that must be reproducible.

Example 7.2 – Simple random sampling

The purpose of this example is to demonstrate the difference between using the RAND() function in Excel and the Random Number Generation feature in the Data Analysis ToolPak. Both tools will be used to draw a random sample of three subjects from the sampling frame of 10 subjects below.

	A	B	C
			Random Number Generator (Uniform
1	Subjects	RAND() results	with seed = 1229)
2	1	0.499401153	0.123661
3	2	0.118153373	0.366435743
4	3	0.21558043	0.663624989
5	4	0.5329594	0.595507675
6	5	0.407077458	0.129734184
7	6	0.426900123	0.63637196
8	7	0.104159091	0.991210669
9	8	0.096211791	0.194586016
10	9	0.885465132	0.604327525
11	10	0.124925856	0.344157231

Example 7.2 – Simple random sampling (*continued*)

Column "B" is populated with the function = rand()

Column "C" is populated by using the following steps:

1. Open the data analysis ToolPak (see tutorial for details)
2. Select "Random Number Generation"

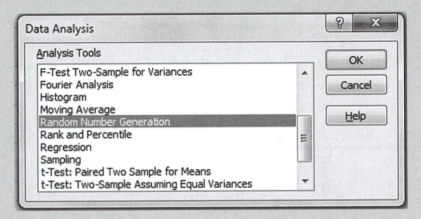

3. Input the number of variables (1), number of random numbers (10), distribution (uniform), random seed (1229), and output range ($C$2)

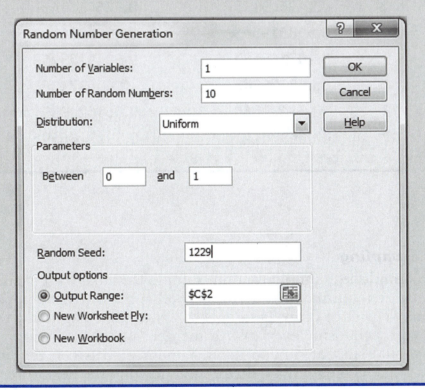

(continued)

Example 7.2 – Simple random sampling (*continued*)

Sort the data range A1:C11 by column C. The first three subjects in the figure below represent the sample. Notice that when the data is sorted by column C the values in column B change. This is because the RAND() function values update each time a recalculation occurs in the spreadsheet. The recalculation is a second reason not to use the RAND() function alone to generate a series of random numbers for sampling, since the sample would not be reproducible by a second analyst.

	A	B	C
	Subjects	RAND() results	Random Number Generator (Uniform with seed = 1229)
1			
2	1	0.674077477	0.123661
3	5	0.571036378	0.129734184
4	8	0.019171959	0.194586016
5	10	0.465559354	0.344157231
6	2	0.149609136	0.366435743
7	4	0.598519545	0.595507675
8	9	0.107165597	0.604327525
9	6	0.662395146	0.63637196
10	3	0.61482544	0.663624989
11	7	0.066374127	0.991210669

Systematic Random Sampling

A **systematic random sample** is a simple random sample that may be generated by selecting every fifth or every tenth member of the sampling frame. If the population includes N members and we wish to draw as sample of size n, then a systemic random sample could be selected by choosing every N/nth member of the population as the sample. The selection should start at random from a member between the first and N/nth member. If N/n is not a whole number, then round down to the next lower whole number to determine the sampling interval. In order to ensure that a systematic random

Example 7.3 – Selecting a systematic random sample

Select a sample of size three from a population of 10 systematic random sampling. $N = 10$, $n = 3$. Select every 10/3 or third member of the population. Select a random number from one to three as the starting point. If three is selected as the random start, then select the third, sixth, and ninth member of the sampling frame.

sample is truly random, the sampling frame should not be sorted in an order that might bias the sample.

Systematic random sampling is a useful tool if the sampling frame is not available electronically. For instance, if a random sample of patients is to be selected from a scanned roster of patients that signed in during one day at a clinic, then the listing of patients serves as the sampling frame and must be keyed into a spreadsheet for sorting. Instead of keying the patient identifiers or sequence numbers into a spreadsheet, systematic random sampling may be used to select the sample directly from the scanned roster.

Stratified Random Sampling

In **stratified random sampling**, the population is divided into similar groups or **strata** based on a set of criteria. Each unit in the population must be assigned to one and only one stratum. Therefore, the strata do not overlap. Once the population is divided into the strata, a simple random sample is selected from each of the strata. The number of units selected from each stratum is typically based on the size of the strata relative to the size of the population.

The estimates derived from stratified random sampling must be weighted by the size of each stratum. The details of analytic techniques required are beyond the scope of this text, but analysts should be aware that the statistical techniques are unique for this sampling design.

Stratified random sampling is appropriate to use when there are subsets of the population that must be included in the analysis or natural separations in the population that might make it more convenient to use this sampling method. For instance, a review of the accuracy of evaluation and management code assignment may be performed using a sample stratified by specialty or clinic site.

Cluster Random Sampling

In **cluster random sampling**, the population is divided into groups before the sample is selected. As in stratified random sampling, the groups or clusters must be mutually exclusive and exhaustive. That is, every unit in the population is assigned to one and

Example 7.4 – Stratified random sample allocation

If a random sample of 90 is selected from a population of evaluation and management visits that are stratified by level, how many should be selected from each stratum? Using a proportional allocation strategy demonstrated below:

Level	Population Count (N)	Percent of Population	Exact Sample Size (n)	Effective Sample Size (n)
1	55	6%	4.95	5
2	183	18%	16.47	16
3	236	24%	21.24	21
4	309	31%	27.81	28
5	217	22%	19.53	20
Totals	1,000	100%	90	90

Note: The exact sample size is typically not an integer. Since only full units can be sampled, the effective sample size is the result of rounding the exact sample size. On occasion, the sum of the effective sample size may not equal the desired sample size due to rounding. If that occurs, it is acceptable to adjust the sample size in a stratum to meet the sample size requirement.

only one cluster. Cluster sampling may be performed as single-stage or two-stage versions. In single-stage cluster sampling, clusters are selected at random and all units in that cluster are included in the sample. An example of single-stage cluster sampling is to randomly select a day in the month and select all cases coded on that day as the sample. In two-stage cluster sampling, the clusters are selected at random and then the units within the randomly selected clusters are selected at random. An example of two-stage cluster sampling is to randomly select three shifts occurring during the month and then randomly select records from the three selected shifts to make up the sample.

Cluster sampling is useful when a sampling frame containing the entire population is not available, but natural groups of the population are available for selection. Care should be taken to ensure that clusters are homogenous. For instance, in the single-stage cluster example where days are selected at random from the month, the analyst may want to exclude weekends from the population of clusters. Specialized data analysis techniques are required to analyze the data resulting from a cluster sample.

Non-Probability Sampling

Convenience Sampling

In **convenience sampling**, the sample is chosen as the name implies: by convenience. Volunteers may be solicited, but all applicants are chosen. Other types of samples that can be used include those samples that are easiest to obtain and those that are available at the lowest cost. A convenience sample is not representative of the entire population.

Judgment Sampling

Judgment sampling is completed by a researcher with expert knowledge of the subject being studied, and choices are made based on the researcher's knowledge base. Data analysts, for example, use judgment sampling when they evaluate data and select records or entries that require further investigation based on their experience.

Analyzing claim histories from a data report is a form of judgment sampling. Judgment sampling allows the analyst to select only the questionable cases for the focused review. Cases should be reviewed for potential coding or sequencing issues, unusually long or short lengths of stay, high total charges, or other issues that do not appear similar to the norm. It should be noted that judgment sampling only establishes that data is questionable and does not establish the accuracy or inaccuracy of the coding or sequencing. Review of the health record documentation is the only process that can determine whether the coding and sequencing are correct or should be changed.

Quota Sampling

Quota sampling segments the population into mutually exclusive groups, as is done in stratified random sampling. Then, judgment sampling is used to select a number of individuals for the sample, such as 50 individuals in each age group of 41–49 and 50–59. This sampling is not a probability sample because judgment is used in the selection of the individual units in the groups. Quota sampling might be used to determine satisfaction with the food in the hospital cafeteria. A researcher might position himself outside the cafeteria and select participants to complete a survey until 10 male and 10 female subjects have completed the survey. The 10 male and 10 female subjects represent the quota. The researcher approaches potential subjects at random, but may be biased toward selecting subjects that appear more approachable and likely to accept the invitation to complete the survey.

Selecting a Judgment Sample for Compliance Monitoring

Using the sample selection techniques and the suggestions found in this chapter, a facility can develop a more effective, focused sample for compliance monitoring. By analyzing the data first, an analyst can create a list of claim histories that should be further reviewed for possible coding or documentation issues. Using this technique helps target the cases that will have changes or highlight areas that need improvement. Using data analysis also allows the analyst to exclude from a focused review those cases that do not appear to have coding or documentation issues.

Selecting a Random Sample Using Statistical Software

RAT-STATS Program from the Office of Inspector General

In addition to selecting a random sample, a data analyst may be asked to determine the appropriate sample size for an audit. The Office of Inspector General (OIG) provides a free statistical program called RAT-STATS that can be used for this purpose (OIG 2007).

The OIG website describes RAT-STATS, developed by the Regional Advanced Techniques Staff (RATS) in San Francisco, California, as a package of statistical software tools designed to assist the user in selecting random samples and evaluating the audit results. The goal behind this program was to create valuable analytical tools that could be easily used by auditors. Windows RAT-STATS 2007, the latest version of RAT-STATS available, includes all programs from the original Disk Operating System (DOS) version for the modern platform (OIG 2007). The program, user guide, and companion guide can all be downloaded from the OIG website (see online appendix G).

The guides that accompany the program provide the analyst with step-by-step instructions in choosing a statistically valid sample at a given confidence level by displaying screen settings and sample report outputs. This is a powerful program that helps ensure that the samples selected will be considered valid by OIG in the event of a government audit.

RAT-STATS – How to Determine an Appropriate Sample Size

The RAT-STATS software supports determining an appropriate sample size for two types of studies:

1. Attribute – studies where the variable of interest is a rate or proportion. Examples include MS-DRG change rates, coding accuracy rates, or complication rates.

2. Variable – studies where the variable of interest is a quantity measured on an interval or ratio scale. Examples include payment error amount, length of stay in a specialty unit, or wait times in an emergency department.

The following sections will demonstrate the steps in determining an appropriate sample size. The screen shots are taken from RAT-STATS 2007.

Figure 7.1 **RAT-STATS opening screen**

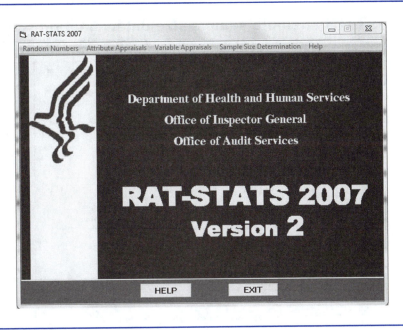

Source: RAT-STATS, 2007.

Figure 7.2 **RAT-STATS sample size determination choices**

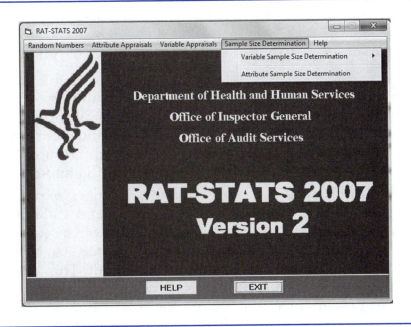

Source: OIG RAT-STATS, 2007.

Attribute Studies

Figure 7.3 RAT-STATS attribute sample size determination screen

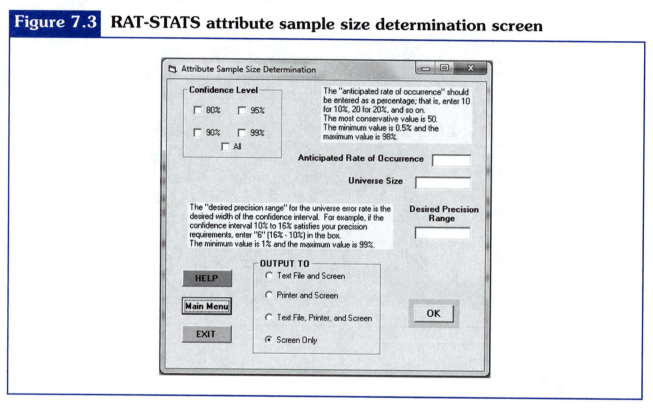

Source: OIG RAT-STATS, 2007.

Selecting a sample for an attribute study requires the selection of the following parameters:

1. Confidence level – The results of the study is typically reported as a confidence interval. For instance, a 95 percent confidence interval for the complication rate is five percent ± one percent. Select the desired confidence level. Click Select All to observe the impact of confidence level on the required sample size. Confidence level and confidence intervals were discussed in both chapters 4 and 5.

2. Anticipated rate of occurrence – Selection of a sample size requires some knowledge of the rate to be expected. Refer back to chapter 4 and notice that the width of the confidence interval for a rate is a function of the rate derived from the sample. This may seem like circular logic, but sample size determination in any study requires some educated guess of the end result. This is sometimes derived from a smaller probe study, previous studies, or rates found in research literature. The most conservative value to use for an attribute study is 50 percent, but 50 percent should only be used if no additional information is available. This value will result in the largest sample size.

3. Universe size – Number of units in the universe.

4. Desired precision range – This is the target width of the confidence interval to be derived from the sample. A wider confidence interval will require a smaller sample size. A narrower confidence interval will require a larger sample size.

Example 7.5 – Attribute sample size determination

Clerical staff enters the physician orders into the computer order entry system at Metro Clinic. Physicians are then required to enter an electronic signature to verify the order. The manager of Metro Clinic is concerned that physicians may not be completing the signature step and wishes to perform an audit. The variable of interest is the presence or absence of the physician's signature, so this is an attribute study. The population size is 8,298 orders from the last fiscal year. The manager requests a data analyst to determine the proper sample size to estimate the rate of missing signatures ± five percent with 95 percent confidence.

The analyst first determines the sample size using 50 percent as the anticipated rate of occurrence:

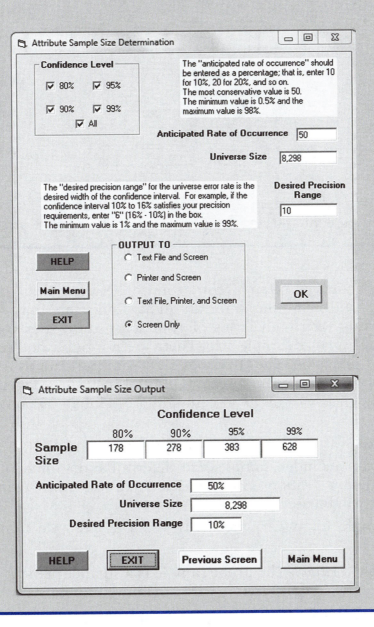

(continued)

Example 7.5 – Attribute sample size determination (*continued*)

The manager is surprised by the sample size required and only has enough funding to review 150 orders. The analyst explains that the sample size is based on setting the anticipated rate of occurrence at 50 percent and asks if the manager has the results of any previous audits that may be used to generate a more accurate sample size. The manager states that the error rate from last year's audit was 15 percent and that may be used as the anticipated rate of occurrence. The analyst regenerates the sample sizes displayed below:

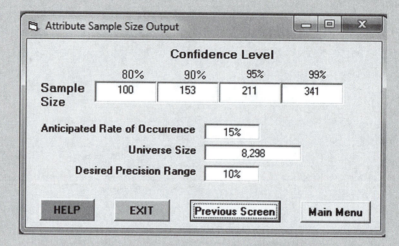

The manager decides to compromise on the confidence level moving it from 95 percent to 90 percent and reviews a random sample of 153 orders.

Sample size selection is often a compromise between desired confidence level, precision, and the budget available for an audit. End users may start by requesting very precise intervals with high levels of confidence until they realize the practical implications of such a large sample size. There are not published rules for the correct confidence level or precision. The OIG does offer some guidance for providers that are subject to a corporate integrity agreement (Office of Inspector General, 2012). The OIG recommends confidence level of 90 percent and precision of 25 percent.

Variable Studies

RAT-STATS software includes sample size determination for a number of variable studies. For this demonstration an unrestricted variable study using a probe sample with no probe file, will be used.

Selecting a sample for a variable study requires the selection of the following parameters:

1. Probe sample format – The probe sample is a smaller pre study that will be used to determine the sample size. As with attribute studies, the width or precision of

Figure 7.4   RAT-STATS variable sample size determination screen

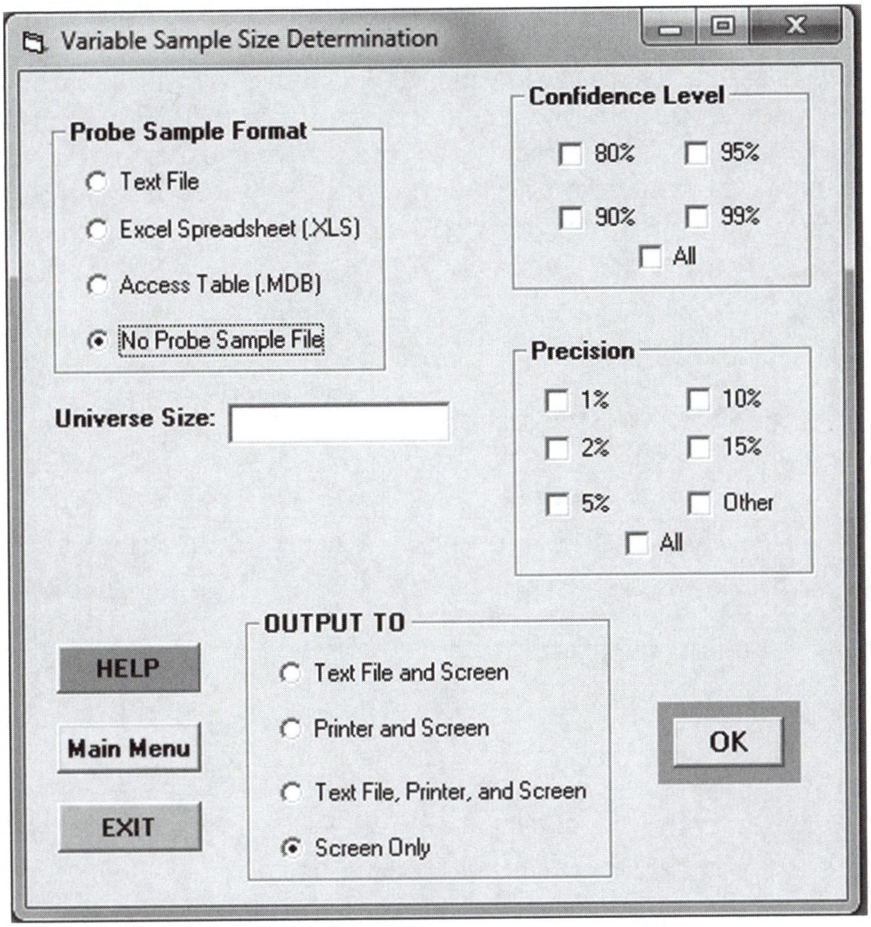

the confidence interval is determined by the standard deviation of the sample. The probe sample will supply an estimate of the standard deviation that may be used to determine the sample size. In this example, no probe sample file is designated. The user is prompted to enter the mean and standard deviation from the probe sample in subsequent steps.

2. Confidence level – Desired confidence level for the reporting of the results.
3. Precision – Width of the confidence interval to be reported.
4. Universe size – The number of units in the population.

Unlike the attribute sample size determination, a probe sample is required for variable sample size determination. The selection of a probe sample is the best method to determine the a prior or estimated standard deviation for the sample. The OIG suggests a probe sample of 50 units, but there a probe sample size may be driven more by budget and time constraints as well.

Example 7.6 – Variable sample size determination

The owner of a clinic wishes to assess the validity of the claims submitted by a particular physician. They fear that the physician may be claiming to visit nursing home patients more often than the documentation may support during 2010. The physician billed 5,753 claims during 2010. A probe study of 15 cases resulted in an average overpayment of $23.69 per case with a standard deviation of $30.98. How large of a sample should be selected to determine a 90 percent confidence interval for the average overpayment per claim with 25 percent precision?

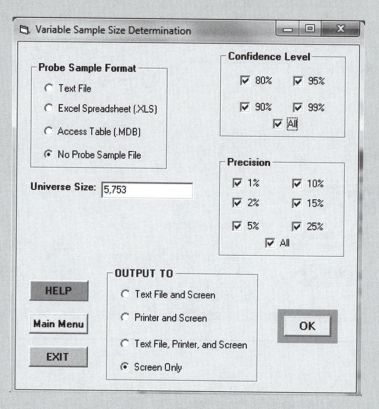

Note: 25 percent is not listed as a default in the precision section. Clicking the "other" checkbox allows the user to enter the value 25 percent.

After clicking OK, the user must enter the mean and standard deviation from the probe sample.

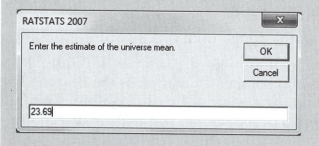

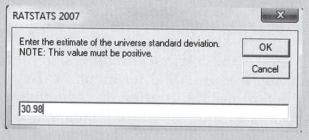

Example 7.6 – Attribute sample size determination (continued)

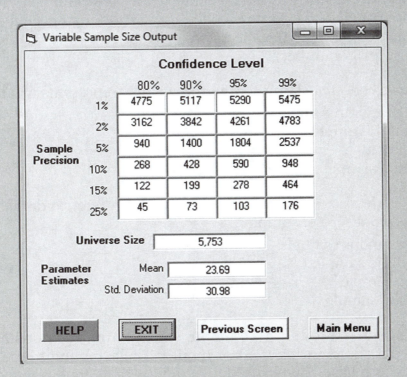

		Confidence Level			
		80%	90%	95%	99%
Sample Precision	1%	4775	5117	5290	5475
	2%	3162	3842	4261	4783
	5%	940	1400	1804	2537
	10%	268	428	590	948
	15%	122	199	278	464
	25%	45	73	103	176

Universe Size   5,753

Parameter Estimates   Mean   23.69
Std. Deviation   30.98

HELP   EXIT   Previous Screen   Main Menu

The sample size for 90 percent confidence level and 25 percent precision is 73. Notice that the sample size increases as the confidence level increases moving across the columns from left to right. The sample size decreases as the precision moves from more precise (one percent) to less precise (25 percent) moving down the rows from top to bottom. Remember that precision is the width of the confidence interval; therefore, a higher value for precision corresponds to the wider, less precise interval.

 # Review Questions

1. A listing of all subjects eligible to be sampled is called:
   a. Sample
   b. Strata
   c. Random number
   d. Sampling frame

2. What information should be included in a sampling plan?
   a. Universe or population
   b. Random seed
   c. Inclusion and exclusion criteria
   d. All of the above

3. Which of the following scenarios represents a non probability sample?
   a. A sample of 10 selected via random number assignment
   b. A sample of the first 10 students entering a classroom
   c. A sample of all of the records coded on a randomly selected date
   d. A sample of the first 10 subjects on a list sorted by the last two digits of their social security number

4. A random selection of claims within three DRGs represents what type of sample?
   a. Simple random sample
   b. Systematic sample
   c. Cluster sample
   d. Stratified sample

5. A random selection of all of the claims within three randomly selected DRGs represents what type of sample?
   a. Simple random sample
   b. Systematic sample
   c. Cluster sample
   d. Stratified sample

6. An analyst is asked to select a random sample from the population of patients that visited a clinic during the last month. The sampling frame is presented to the analyst as a hard copy list. What sampling technique is more appropriate in this situation?
   a. Simple random sample
   b. Systematic sample
   c. Cluster sample
   d. Stratified sample

7. Why is setting and recording the random seed important in random number generation?
   a. All random number generation programs require a seed
   b. The random numbers will be reproducible
   c. The sample is not random unless the seed is set
   d. The random seed is not important in sampling

8. RAT-STATS is:
   a. A sampling software tool distributed by the OIG
   b. A procedure in Statistical Analysis System
   c. A function in the Excel Data Toolpak
   d. A practice dataset for statisticians

9. Which of the following represents an attribute study?
   a. Estimate the amount of overpayment at a clinic
   b. Estimate the DRG change rate after documentation queries
   c. Estimate the length of stay for the typical CHF patient
   d. Estimate the number of claim denials at a hospital

10. What impact does increasing the sample size have on precision?

    a. Larger sample size results in a less precise estimate
    b. Large sample sizes result in a more precise estimate
    c. Sample size does not impact precision

📖 References

CMS. 2011. *Medicare Program Integrity Manual Chapter 8 – Administrative Actions and Statistical Sampling for Overpayment Estimates*. Baltimore: CMS.

Office of Inspector General (OIG). 2012. Corporate Integrity Agreement FAQ. https://oig.hhs.gov/faqs/corporate-integrity-agreements-faq.asp

Office of Inspector General (OIG). 2007. RAT-STATS - Statistical Software. http://oig.hhs.gov/compliance/rat-stats/index.asp

Osborn, C.E. 2006. *Statistical Applications for Health Information Management*, 2nd ed. Sudbury: Jones and Bartlett Publishers.

Exploratory Data Applications

KEY TERMS

Case Mix Index

Data mining

Exploratory data analysis (EDA)

Hospital-acquired condition (HAC)

Exploratory data analysis (EDA) is used regularly in the healthcare setting to find trends and patterns in the various data sources available for analysis. EDA is sometimes called **data mining**. EDA is primarily performed using descriptive statistics. Patterns or aberrations found in the data may be further investigated using random sampling and statistical inference. This chapter includes a number of examples of how EDA and descriptive statistics are used in healthcare operations.

Diagnosis-Related Groups (DRGs) Data Analysis

Case Mix Index (CMI) Analysis

A common way to aggregate data about MS-DRGs is to calculate the **Case Mix Index (CMI)** for all discharges or other meaningful groupings of discharges. The CMI is the average of all DRG weights assigned during a period of time. This average provides an index of the Medicare Severity Diagnostic Related Groups (MS-DRG) frequencies by relative weight, providing one number that displays meaningful information about the patient mix treated by a hospital.

The CMI, which describes the patient population in a single number as well as the average revenue per case when it is multiplied by the hospital's Medicare or commercial payer base rate, can be tracked over time and between facilities. While the CMI technically only refers to Medicare patients, some facilities calculate the CMI and DRG for all patients to provide a consistent, measurable, and relative intensive weight for the entire population served.

Calculating the Case Mix Index

To calculate the CMI from the volume of cases by MS-DRG, calculate the weighted average MS-DRG weight by completing these steps:

1. Multiply the number of discharges in each MS-DRG by the relative weight of that MS-DRG.
2. Sum the relative weights from step 1.
3. Sum the number of discharges in the MS-DRGs chosen to be evaluated.
4. Divide the total relative weights from step 2 by the total number of discharges from step 3.

Table 8.1 shows the case mix calculation for a select group of MS-DRGs.

Table 8.1 Case mix calculation

MS-DRG	Cases	Relative Weight	Total Relative Weight
181	10	1.2108	12.108
192	16	0.7072	11.315
286	20	2.0617	41.234
287	27	1.0709	28.914
615	2	1.4036	2.807
644	3	1.0508	3.152
657	4	1.9904	7.962
	82		107.493
		107.493/82 =	1.311
Case mix index =			1.311

Table 8.2 shows the comparison of two hospitals for both Medicare patients and the entire patient population for the four quarters of fiscal year 2010 (FY10).

Table 8.2 Case mix index comparison report

	1st qtr FY10	2nd qtr FY10	3rd qtr FY10	4th qtr FY10
Hospital A				
Medicare patients	1.68	1.58	1.73	1.67
All patients	1.49	1.43	1.51	1.47
Hospital B				
Medicare patients	1.26	1.29	1.38	1.35
All patients	1.13	1.14	1.10	1.19

Monitoring Case Mix

The CMI should be monitored over time, using a valid baseline to help track any deviations. "The average relative weight, percentages of discharges by specialty, average length of stay (ALOS), and average charges are used to validate an organization's CMI, which affects the calculation for each DRG payment" (Hanna 2002).

Facilities should ask questions about whether the CMI is steady, whether it increases steadily or drastically, or whether it decreases in a sharp or sudden decline (Casto and Forrestal 2012, 45). Answers to these questions can help frame the intensity of the review that needs to take place regarding CMI changes. Many facilities use a threshold of a 2 percent change, either positive or negative, in a given period as the trigger for comprehensive evaluation.

When tracking the CMI over long periods of time, it should also be remembered that the DRG system changes from year to year. To allow appropriate comparisons, the DRGs and codes from one year must be mapped, or translated, to the new DRGs and codes for the next year in the DRG grouper, and then both sets of data must be regrouped using this updated grouper (Wozniak 2002).

The CMI can also be calculated and tracked by the 25 major diagnostic categories (MDCs) into which all MS-DRGs are divided. Most MDCs are based on body systems and include diseases and disorders relating to a particular system. However, some MDCs, such as burns, involve multiple organ systems. Of interest would be the MDC with the highest CMI over time (Bryant 2008). Tracking the index by the MDC can help pinpoint which areas are increasing or decreasing.

Table five from the inpatient prospective payment system (IPPS) Final Rule for FY13 can be found on the CMS website (see online appendix G). This file provides the listing of the MS-DRGs that are assigned to each MDC as well as the complete title of each MS-DRG, the relative weight, the geometric mean length of stay (with outliers and transfer cases removed), and the arithmetic mean length of stay.

Hospitals can also monitor MS-DRGs using several other methods and measures. Facilities can compare the percentage of discharges in each of the MS-DRG severity groupings, the payment amount against the range of charges for the discharges in each MS-DRG, or the length of stay for the discharges in each MS-DRG. These comparisons can be done with either the Medical Provider Analysis and Review (MEDPAR) data discussed in chapter 2 or other comparative data available to the facility.

Other MS-DRG Measures

A facility's population, or case mix, can be analyzed by measuring MS-DRGs in other ways. For example, to analyze the severity of illness of the population, the percentage of patients in each of the MS-DRG pairs or triplets and the percentage of the overall population that has a complication or comorbidity (CC) or major complication or comorbidity (MCC) is vital information. A complication is a medical condition that arises during an inpatient hospitalization, such as a postoperative wound infection. A comorbidity is a preexisting condition that, because of its presence with a specific diagnosis, causes an increase in length of stay by at least one day in approximately 75 percent of the cases. A major complication/comorbidity is the most severe of complications or comorbidities that place a patient in the highest-severity category within the MS-DRG system.

MS-DRG Pair or Triplet Comparison

Facilities should determine the percentage of patients discharged within each of the different severity levels of each MS-DRG. Comparing the facility percentages to national percentages can help determine whether a facility's documentation should be examined for deficiencies or whether its patient population is somehow different from the national average. For example, if the facility percentage in a higher-weighted MS-DRG is high because the facility has a nationally known transplant surgeon on staff that specializes in high-risk transplants, this should show in the facility's MS-DRG percentages.

Calculating the Pair or Triplet Percentage

The percentage of discharges in a particular MS-DRG member of a pair is calculated as:

$$\% \text{ of CC Cases} = \frac{n(\text{CC MS} - \text{DRG})}{n(\text{CC MS} - \text{DRG}) + n(\text{no CC MS} - \text{DRG})} \times 100$$

where "*n*" = the number of discharges in that MS-DRG. If there are three MS-DRGs in a grouping (triplet), add the totals of all three MS-DRGs for the denominator.

$$\% \text{ of CC Cases} = \frac{n(\text{CC MS} - \text{DRG})}{n(\text{MCC MS} - \text{DRG}) + n(\text{CC MS} - \text{DRG}) + n(\text{no CC MS} - \text{DRG})} \times 100$$

$$\% \text{ of MCC Cases} = \frac{n(\text{MCC MS} - \text{DRG})}{n(\text{MCC MS} - \text{DRG}) + n(\text{CC MS} - \text{DRG}) + n(\text{no CC MS} - \text{DRG})} \times 100$$

Example 8.1 – MCC percentage

Calculate the MCC case percentage for the following MS-DRG Pair:

MS-DRG 595, Major skin disorders with MCC, relative wt. 1.3997, 1st qtr FY08 volume = 8

MS-DRG 596, Major skin disorders without MCC, relative wt. 0.8766, 1st qtr FY08 volume = 22

$$\text{Percent of MCC Cases} = \frac{n(\text{MCC MS} - \text{DRG})}{n(\text{MCC MS} - \text{DRG}) + n(\text{no MCC MS} - \text{DRG})} \times 100$$

$$= \frac{8}{22 + 8} \times 100 = 26.7\%$$

Overall, 90 percent of all MS-DRGs are affected by the presence of a complication or comorbidity or major complication or comorbidity, with 61 percent of the MS-DRGs having triplets and 29 percent having pairs. Therefore, calculating and tracking the percentages in pairs or triplets as well as the CC or MCC capture rate is very important to understanding the severity of illness and the CMI of the patient population.

Complication or Comorbidity (CC) and Major Complication or Comorbidity (MCC) Capture Rate

The CC capture rate is the number of patients with CCs compared to all of the patients in the population. With the changes in the CC list and the addition of MCCs in the MS-DRG system, facilities are finding that the CC capture rate is much lower than it had been previously, and new benchmarks need to be established for MS-DRGs.

The CC capture rate is a valuable tool in measuring the overall severity of patients served by the facility as a whole or by a particular physician or specialty. Assuming that the coding is accurately completed, the rate can help measure the specificity of physician documentation.

Calculating the CC or MCC Capture Rate

The CC or MCC capture rate is calculated using the following formula, where n equals the number of discharges in that MS-DRG:

$$\text{CC / MCC Capture Rate} = \frac{n(\text{all CC MS} - \text{DRG}) + n(\text{all MCC MS} - \text{DRG})}{n(\text{all MS} - \text{DRG})} \times 100$$

To calculate the CC capture rate separately, use the following formula:

$$\text{CC Capture Rate} = \frac{n(\text{all CC MS} - \text{DRG})}{n(\text{all CC MS} - \text{DRG})} \times 100$$

For the MCC capture rate, use the following formula:

$$\text{MCC Capture Rate} = \frac{n(\text{all MCC MS} - \text{DRG})}{n(\text{all MS} - \text{DRG})} \times 100$$

MS-DRG Payments Versus Charges or Length of Stay

Hospitals frequently look at MS-DRG data for comparisons between payments and charges or geometric mean length of stay and actual length of stay. This data can be used to analyze whether to increase or decrease program offerings within a hospital or health system. In addition, length-of-stay inconsistencies, along with a low CC or MCC capture rate, can indicate where coding and documentation education should be targeted regarding a particular MS-DRG, for a department, or for a physician.

Methods of MS-DRG Analysis

Many facilities set a threshold for change in the case mix that requires analysis. A common threshold is a 2 percent change in either direction, with a drop of more than 5 percent being a critical value.

Analyzing changes in case mix requires reports that categorize data in specific enough detail to reveal where and when the change in case mix has occurred (Wozniak 2002). The most useful starting point is frequency reports listing all of the cases by MS-DRG for the period (month or quarter). By comparing the number of cases in each MS-DRG over several periods, significant increases or decreases can be pinpointed. Even a small change in the number of cases in a highly weighted MS-DRG can cause a change in the case mix.

When an MS-DRG is found that explains a significant difference in the case mix, case mix data should be compared with and without the MS-DRG to determine if the issue persists. If MS-DRG frequency reports do not provide an explanation for a change in case mix, other reports should be used to search for other areas of change. Diagnosis and procedure frequency reports, as described in chapter 4, may also help explain a change. Physician reports or service reports showing admission numbers may also be used.

The data analyst should routinely ask the administrative team to maintain a list of changes or brainstorm additions or deletions to an existing listing for use in explaining a change in case mix. A list of changes might include items such as:

- Seasonality: flu season, pneumonia season, patient movement in or out of the area based on weather, arrival of new residents in July
- Changes in an area's healthcare environment: opening or closing a significant service line, adding new equipment, a new hospital, loss of a hospital in the service area
- Medical staff changes: loss or gain of physicians associated with high relative weight MS-DRGs
- Medicare contracting changes: contracting changes with Medicare managed-care plans versus Medicare fee-for-service plans (Wilson and Dunn 2009).

To this list, the management staff for the coding function might add information about:

- Changes in coding: significant changes in coding rules related to the way MS-DRGs are assigned to a major service lines
- Stability of the coding staff: new coding staff or a change in coding assignments that could cause variability in code assignments.

In addition, facilities may plan to track CMI data with and without the MS-DRG data on a new program. For example, a facility develops a new lung transplant program and tracks the CMI with and without MS-DRG 007, lung transplants for a minimum of several years. By doing so, the facility can make consistent comparisons of the case mix over time while still being able to determine the change in the case mix with the inclusion of the new program. Figure 8.1 shows the comparison of the case mix with and without the lung transplant program, started in the second quarter of FY12.

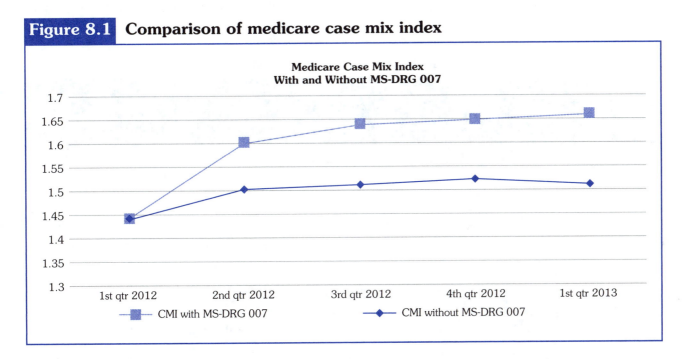

Figure 8.1 **Comparison of medicare case mix index**

Other Factors Influencing MS-DRGs

Since the implementation of the original DRG system in the 1980s, hospitals have had the potential to receive additional payments when complications occurred during the course of a patient's hospitalization. This concept of paying extra for potentially preventable complications has been challenged during the past few years and has led to the implementation of the present on admission (POA) indicator to identify those conditions that arose following the admission. When a condition is not POA, it is termed a hospital-acquired condition and will not be included in the calculation to increase the level of MS-DRG severity, beginning October 1, 2008. A **hospital-acquired condition (HAC)** is a condition that is not present at the time of inpatient admission, results in the assignment of the case to a DRG that has a higher payment when the condition is present as a secondary diagnosis, and could reasonably have been prevented through application of evidence-based guidelines.

Present on Admission (POA) Indicator

For discharges occurring on or after October 1, 2008, hospitals do not receive additional payment for cases in which a condition on the HAC list was not POA. That is, the case would be paid as though the secondary diagnosis were not present. Note that if the HAC was the only CC or MCC associated with the case, this CC or MCC would not be used in the calculation of the MS-DRG, and the payment would not be increased. However, if other CC or MCCs are associated with the case, the higher MS-DRG would be assigned, and the payment would be higher.

The POA indicators, their descriptions, and the effect on payment are provided in table 8.3.

Table 8.3 Present on admission indicator and the effect on payment

Present on Admission Indicator	Indicator Description	Effect on Payment
Y	Diagnosis was present at time of inpatient admission.	CMS will pay the CC or MCC DRG for those selected HACs that are coded as "Y" for the POA indicator.
N	Diagnosis was not present at time of impatient admission.	CMS will not pay the CC or MCC DRG for those selected HACs that are coded as "N" for the POA indicator.
U	Documentation insufficient to determine if the condition was present at the time of inpatient admission.	CMS will not pay the CC or MCC DRG for those selected HACs that are coded as "U" for the POA indicator.
W	Provider unable to clinically determine whether the condition was present at the time of inpatient admission.	CMS will pay the CC or MCC DRG for those selected HACs that are coded as "W" for the POA indicator.
1	Unreported or not used. Exempt from POA reporting. (This code is equivalent to a blank on the UB-04; however, it was determined that blanks are undesirable when submitting this data via the 4010A electronic claim.)	Does not affect payment. All POA indicator options coded as "1" are exempt from the HAC payment provision.

Not all hospitals are currently required by Centers for Medicare and Medicaid Services (CMS) to submit the POA indicator. Critical access hospitals, long-term care hospitals, inpatient rehabilitation facilities, inpatient psychiatric facilities, cancer hospitals, children's inpatient hospitals, and hospitals in Maryland operating under waivers are exempt from POA reporting and the HAC payment provision. However, some states have POA reporting requirements that have been in effect for years and these may apply to a different set of reporting facilities.

The HAC that affect payment by CMS for FY13 include:

- Foreign object retained after surgery
- Air embolism

- Blood incompatibility
- Stages III and IV pressure ulcers
- Falls and trauma
  - Fractures
  - Dislocations
  - Intracranial injuries
  - Crushing injuries
  - Burns
  - Other injuries

- Catheter-associated urinary tract infection (UTI)
- Vascular catheter-associated infection
- Manifestations of poor glycemic control
  - Diabetic ketoacidosis
  - Nonketotic hyperomolar coma
  - Secondary diabetes with ketoacidosis
  - Secondary diabetes with hyperosmolarity

- Surgical site infection-mediastinitis after a coronary artery bypass graft (CABG)
- Surgical site infection following certain orthopedic procedures
  - Spine
  - Neck
  - Shoulder
  - Elbow

- Surgical site infection following bariatric surgery for obesity
  - Laparoscopic gastric bypass
  - Gastronenterostomy
  - Laparoscopic gastric restrictive surgery

- Surgical site infection following cardiac implantable electronic device (CIED)
- Deep vein thrombosis and pulmonary embolism following certain orthopedic procedures
  - Total knee replacement
  - Hip replacement

- Iatrogenic pneumothorax with venous catheterization
  (CMS 2012)

To determine the potential impact on a facility, the data analyst would analyze those HAC that were coded the same way in past years to determine the extent of potential lost revenue. The analyst would also attempt to determine the impact of coding changes made for the current fiscal year on future payment rates by tracking HACs that may be excluded from payment in the future.

Other Diagnosis-Related Group Methodologies

All-Patient Diagnosis-Related Groups (AP-DRGs)

In 1987, New York asked 3M Health Information Systems to enhance the DRG system to cover all non-Medicare patients including children and neonates. In response, 3M developed the all-patient diagnosis-related group (AP-DRG) system. This system is in use by some states as the basis of their Medicaid payment systems and can also be referred to as the "New York Grouper."

All-Patient Refined Diagnosis-Related Groups (APR-DRGs)

The AP-DRG system was later enhanced to include severity of illness and risk of mortality of patients. This next generation of DRGs became known as all-patient refined DRGs (APR-DRGs) and included four subclasses within each base DRG that divided patients into groups by severity and risk of mortality. APR-DRGs remove all age, CC, and MCC groupings and substitute two sets of four subclasses: one group of four subclasses for severity and one group of four subclasses for risk of mortality. During the group assignment process, the APR-DRG system divides APR-DRGs into major diagnostic using a method similar to that used in MS-DRGs.

The complete title of an APR-DRG contains the base APR-DRG (for example: 225 Appendectomy), a digit from 1–4 to describe severity, and a digit from 1–4 to describe the risk of mortality; the three components are separated by dashes. The rankings for both severity and mortality are:

1 = Minor
2 = Moderate
3 = Major
4 = Extreme

Therefore, the appendectomy grouping with the lowest severity and risk is 225-1-1, while the grouping with the highest severity and risk is 225-4-4. Each APR-DRG has a relative weight assigned that reflects the severity of illness and risk of mortality for patients assigned to that category.

It should be noted that the relative weight assigned to an APR-DRG group has no relationship to the relative weight assigned to an MS-DRG. MS-DRG relative weights are based on the resource intensity measured as the cost to care a Medicare paitent assigned to the category. These two weighting systems are completely separate and are scaled based on different mesures of resource intensity.

Case Mix Index for APR-DRGs

The CMI for APR-DRGs tells the same story as the CMI for MS-DRGs and is calculated the same way. In addition to tracking the overall CMI, facilities may want to track the index by MDC or the case mix for all of the subclasses of one particular APR-DRG. For example, the facility that developed a new lung transplant program with MS-DRG data depicted in figure 8.1 also tracks patient severity by using APR-DRGs. Further, the facility might want to track the CMI for APR-DRG 002, Heart and Lung Transplant, over time to determine the severity of its cases. Table 8.4 shows the calculation of the CMI for this APR-DRG in FY08.

Table 8.4 **Case mix calculation for APR-DRG 002**

Heart and/or Lung Transplant (FY08)			
APR-DRG	Cases	Rel wt	Total wt
002-1	2	11.1398	22.2796
002-2	3	12.1994	36.5982
002-3	1	18.3022	18.3022
002-4	1	27.2380	27.238
			104.418
	7	104.418/7 =	14.9169
Case mix index =			14.9169

Ambulatory Patient Classification (APC) Data Analysis

Ambulatory patient classifications (APCs) are the groups used by CMS to categorize and pay for hospital outpatient visits under the hospital outpatient prospective payment system (HOPPS). There can be more than one APC group associated with an outpatient visit or a one-to-many relationship. Therefore, APC analysis can be more challenging than the MS-DRG analysis, where a one-to-one relationship exists between an MS-DRG and the discharge.

Challenges in APC Analysis

APC analysis is challenging not only because of the one-to-many relationship of outpatient visits to APCs, but also because CMS makes many changes every year to the APC groupings. This causes a lack of consistency from year to year, making it more difficult to interpret trends and patterns from one year to the next.

The 2013 HOPPS Final Rule is Regulation Number CMS-1589-FC, available on the CMS website (see online appendix G). The file entitled "Median Costs for Hospital Outpatient Services, by HCPCS code" gives the outpatient current procedural terminology (CPT) and Healthcare Common Procedure Coding System (HCPCS) code volumes, and the file entitled "Median Costs for Hospital Outpatient Services, by ambulatory payment classification (APC) group" gives the outpatient volumes by APC code. Appendix C of the Final Rule lists all of the payable CPT and HCPCS codes, grouped by APC, including relative weights and payment rates. Final rule documents from prior years are also available on the CMS website. These documents would help the data analyst determine which services are associated with which APC in any given year and would help build reports that can better track this data over time.

APC Frequency Reports

Frequency (or volume) reports are listings of codes or groups and the associated number of times a particular code or group has been assigned during a specific time frame. These basic reports provide the data for simple analysis and the bell curve discussion found later in this chapter. Table 8.5 shows the APC data associated with hospital clinic visits, emergency visits, and critical care services for calendar year 2012 from a sample hospital and the most recent comparative data from the Medicare Final Rule for 2013. This table was developed using the files listed above.

Table 8.5 APC frequency report for my local hospital in MyTown, TX

APC	APC Short Descriptor	SI	Relative Weight	Payment Rate	Facility APC Volume 2012	Total Payments	Medicare National Volume 2011
604	Level 1 hospital clinic visits	V	0.796	$56.77	12,187	$691,856	5,143,728
605	Level 2 hospital clinic visits	V	1.0332	$73.68	15,233	$1,122,367	10,900,345
606	Level 3 hospital clinic visits	V	1.3596	$96.96	27,420	$2,658,643	4,210,813
607	Level 4 hospital clinic visits	V	1.8017	$128.48	30,467	$3,914,400	997,979
608	Level 5 hospital clinic visits	V	2.465	$175.79	16,249	$2,856,412	172,002
609	Level 1 emergency visits	V	0.7266	$51.82	540	$27,983	342,630
613	Level 2 emergency visits	V	1.2923	$92.16	2,698	$248,648	1,252,945
614	Level 3 emergency visits	V	2.0103	$143.36	4,857	$696,300	4,366,407
615	Level 4 emergency visits	V	3.2164	$229.37	3,068	$703,707	4,736,990
616	Level 5 emergency visits	V	4.8338	$344.71	2,428	$836,956	2,920,948

Methods of Analysis

A report similar to table 8.5 is helpful in analyzing any type of data but is particularly helpful for APCs. For APCs that have not had a number change or a change in the associated CPT and HCPCS codes, yearly trending can be done. When a reimbursement change is announced, future revenue projections can be done by substituting new payment rates for previous payment rates.

APC Service-Mix Index (SMI)

The service-mix index describes the outpatient population in a single number. The index for outpatient services paid under APCs is calculated using the same method used to calculate the CMI. The service-mix index for My Local Hospital in MyTown, TX, displayed in table 8.5, is 1.6754 and is calculated in table 8.6.

Table 8.6 **Servive-mix index calculation for my local hospital in MyTown, TX**

APC	APC Short Descriptor	SI	Relative Weight	Facility APC Volume 2012	Total Weight
604	Level 1 hospital clinic visits	V	0.796	12,187	9,701
605	Level 2 hospital clinic visits	V	1.0332	15,233	15,739
606	Level 3 hospital clinic visits	V	1.3596	27,420	37,280
607	Level 4 hospital clinic visits	V	1.8017	30,467	54,892
608	Level 5 hospital clinic visits	V	2.465	16,249	40,054
609	Level 1 emergency visits	V	0.7266	540	392
613	Level 2 emergency visits	V	1.2923	2,698	3,487
614	Level 3 emergency visits	V	2.0103	4,857	9,764
615	Level 4 emergency visits	V	3.2164	3,068	9,868
616	Level 5 emergency visits	V	4.8338	2,428	11,736
	Totals			115,147	192,913
	APC Service Mix Index (SMI)				1.6754

Outpatient Code Editor (OCE) Codes

The integrated Outpatient Code Editor (OCE) software used by Medicare to assign APCs to outpatient claims also reports edit codes when the claim cannot be successfully processed. These codes were previously discussed in chapter 2 in relation to the patient accounts system and information about the outcomes of the claims submission process.

When these edit codes are analyzed for commonality and organized by frequency, they lend clues to problems within the outpatient claims processing system. Consider the following two examples.

Example one: A large number of occurrences of Edit 21, Medical visit on the same day as a type T or S procedure without modifier 25, would indicate that failure to attach the 25 modifier to services provided in certain locations is causing line item rejections of clinic or emergency department visit codes.

Example two: Edit 28, Code not recognized by Medicare; alternate code for same service may be available, might indicate that the item is set up incorrectly in the Chargemaster.

The complete listing of these codes and their descriptions can be found on the CMS website (see online appendix G).

Charge Analysis

APC analysis is often performed to look for missing charges. It is accomplished by analyzing the consistency in the data. Reports designed to display data by primary APC (the highest-weighted APC) and any associated APCs for that encounter tell the analyst which procedures are commonly grouped together. When these groupings of procedures are not found in some of the cases, the analyst becomes suspicious and investigates further for possible missing-charge patterns.

APC analysis can also be done in reverse by designing reports to display revenue codes that are submitted without CPT and HCPCS codes, thereby looking for services that are not being entered correctly or are not set up correctly in the Chargemaster.

For example, St. Anywhere Health System implemented a flu and pneumovax clinic for the first time this year. Business Services reports a large increase in the number of return to provider (RTP) OCE edits received from Medicare, specifically Edit 48, Revenue code requires HCPCS. Upon investigation, the data analyst finds these cases to be related to Revenue Code 0636, Drugs requiring detailed coding.

The data in table 8.7 represent the first report developed during the analysis.

Table 8.7 APC0 350, administration of flu and PPV vaccine

	Rev Code 0636 Cases	Rev Code 0636 With HCPCS Code	Rev Code 0636 Without HCPCS Code
Hospital 1	268	268	0
Hospital 2	329	328	1
Hospital 3	211	0	211
Hospital 4	259	259	0

Hospital 3 accounts for the large increase in Edit 48 (RTP). As a next step, the analyst might determine which CPT code or codes are missing and whether the problem is with the chargemaster or with data entry.

Analyzing Patterns of Care

Any pattern of care that has a potential relationship can be analyzed. For example, when analyzing coding patterns in the emergency department (ED), the analyst may evaluate cases in which patients were assigned to APC 0616, Level 5 ED visit, and APC 0617, critical care, but were not admitted. Through the evaluation, the analyst can attempt to determine the reasons why the patients were not admitted. Logic would seem to state that the sickest of all patients presenting to the emergency department would have resulted in inpatient admission, with the exception of patients who expired in the emergency department.

Conversely, the analyst may evaluate cases in which patients were assigned to APC 0609, Level 1 ED visit, and APC 0613, Level 2 ED visit, and were admitted, attempting to determine the reasons for admission. Logic would seem to state that these patients likely would have been discharged home following their treatment in the emergency department.

Other analyses regarding services that are likely performed together could be undertaken, such as looking for a positive correlation between the number of additional APCs associated with APCs 0609, 0613, 0614, 0615, and 0616 as the ED service level increases.

Utilization Pattern Analysis (Bell Curve Graphs)

Bell Curve Analysis

Bell curve analysis can be used to compare and display any group of data that has two or more points. This type of analysis is most commonly used in healthcare to display physician Evaluation and Management (E/M) code percentages but can also be used to compare facility E/M frequencies and MS-DRG data on pairs and triplets.

Steps in Creating a Bell Curve Graph

Obtain data to be used in creating the bell curve graph from internal sources, external sources, or both. Remember to compare data that is related. For example, remember to compare new-patient visits only to each other and not to established-patient visits, and do not group new-patient visits with established-patient visits. For purposes of this discussion, consider an example in which a data analyst looks at the bell curve for Dr. X's practice and the internal medicine (specialty 11) data from Part B utilization data from FY06.

Use a graphing program such as Microsoft Excel and display the data in rows and columns similar to what appears in the following table:

New Patient Visits	Dr. X	Specialty 11 Internal Medicine
99201	24	14,530
99202	60	114,817
99203	288	493,059
99204	228	687,391
99205	36	339,591
Total	636	1,649,388

Convert the physician's volume data and the comparative data in each series to percentages of the whole to determine the percentage of use for each code. The data should look like this:

New Patient Visits	Dr. X	Specialty 11 Internal Medicine
99201	4%	1%
99202	9%	7%
99203	45%	30%
99204	36%	42%
99205	6%	20%

Using the graphing features of the Excel program, create a line graph or bar graph that shows the relationship between Dr. X and the new-patient visits approved by Medicare for payment for internal medicine. The line graph should look like the one in figure 8.2. The choice of line graph versus bar graph is based on personal preference of the analyst or the recipients of the data.

Figure 8.2 **New patient bell curve for Dr. X**

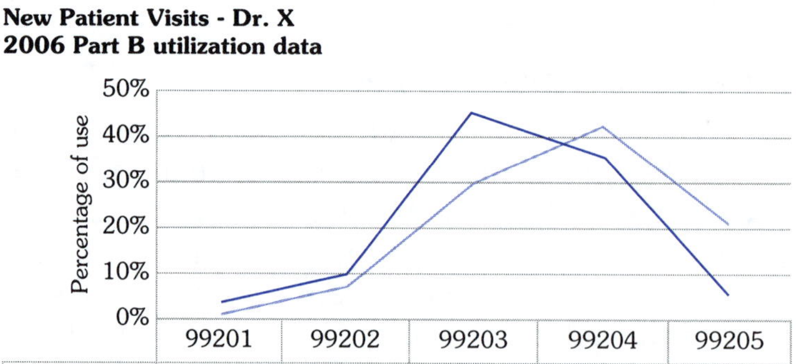

New Patient Visits - Dr. X
2006 Part B utilization data

	99201	99202	99203	99204	99205
Dr.X	4%	9%	45%	36%	6%
Medicare	1%	7%	30%	42%	21%

Dr. X has 15 percent more 99203 visits than the Medicare average and 14 percent fewer 99205 visits than the Medicare comparative data. In general, Dr. X's coding appears to be lower than the Medicare comparative data (the bell curve is shifted to the left), and further analysis should be considered.

Specialty-Specific Graphs for Physician Data

Not all specialties have the same curve. Try graphing the New Patient Visits for Endocrinology (specialty 46) from the Part B utilization data, and the comparative data will show a right shift with percentages of zero percent, three percent, 16 percent, 47 percent, and 34 percent. This shift is because patients who are new to Endocrinology are frequently much more ill than patients who are new to Internal Medicine.

Bell Curves for MS-DRG Data

Bell curves can be created to display the percentage of cases in each division of an MS-DRG pair or triplet. During the development and implementation of the MS-DRG system for FY08, CMS reanalyzed past DRG data using the new version 25 of the MS-DRG grouper. CMS did this reanalysis to determine how past cases would translate into the new MS-DRG system. Table 10 of the Final Rule for IPPS FY09 provides the number of cases that would have been assigned to each MS-DRG using version 26 of the MS-DRG grouper (see online appendix G). Table 10 of the Final Rule for FY13 is based on the FY11 MEDPAR files.

Figure 8.3 provides a comparison of hospital Y and the information provided in table 10 of the Final Rule using version 26 of the MS-DRG grouper for MS-DRGs 034–036, Carotid Artery Stent Procedures.

Figure 8.3 **MS-DRG bell curve for hospital Y**

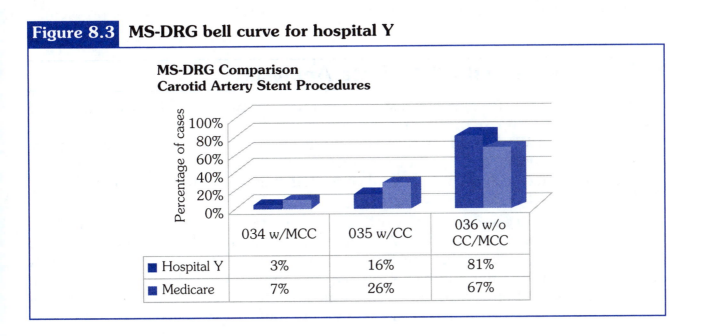

	034 w/MCC	035 w/CC	036 w/o CC/MCC
Hospital Y	3%	16%	81%
Medicare	7%	26%	67%

Methods of Analysis

It is important to remember that the bell curve is a display of the coded data. Therefore, if the bell curve does not resemble the curve found in the comparative data, it does not automatically mean there is a problem. It does mean that there *may* be a problem, however, and further analysis is highly recommended.

Validation of Utilization Patterns

It is always best to carefully determine if the correct comparative data is being used when analyzing physician data. One reason is that many internists develop specialized skills during their years of practicing medicine. Their practice may tend to concentrate on a subspecialty such as Pulmonary Medicine, Endocrinology, or Nephrology, without any change in their credentialing status with Medicare or other insurers. Only a thorough discussion with the physician and analysis of diagnosis frequencies, discussed previously in chapter 4, can determine if the physician's data would be more appropriately compared to data from one of these subspecialties.

In addition, the analyst should determine which types of patients the physician sees. For example, a physician who does not schedule appointments but rather sees only unscheduled, urgent patients may have far more 99213 and 99214 visits than a peer group. Conversely, another physician may use a nurse practitioner to see follow-up patients or those with minor illnesses; the physician personally sees only the sickest patients. This second physician may have a higher than average number of 99214 and 99215 visits, with a bell curve that looks inappropriate. However, if the documentation supports the care of these sicker patients, this bell curve is appropriate.

If a thorough assessment of the variables does not explain the difference in the curves, a comparison of the coded data and the health record documentation should be undertaken. If, after comparison, the documentation matches the codes that were assigned and the services were reasonable and necessary, there is no actual problem.

Relative Value Unit (RVU) Data Analysis

A relative value unit (RVU) is a measure of resource intensity that is assigned to CPT codes. The units compare the relative difficulty and costs associated with the different procedures. An RVU is actually a combination of three subunits that describe the physician work (wRVU), the practice expense (peRVU), and the malpractice expense (mRVU) associated with each individual code. Together, these three subunits make up the Total RVU, or tRVU.

While RVUs are used to evaluate work volumes, patterns, and expenses in physician practices, hospitals can also use RVU values to better quantify work performed by the outpatient service lines that are coded using CPT codes. For example, day surgery statistics may include the number of procedures, the total length of operating room time, and the RVUs for the procedures performed. Each statistic tells a slightly different story about the work performed in the day surgery unit.

In radiology, managers use RVUs to "measure productivity using historical data to derive meaningful benchmarks by removing subjectivity such as differences in work habits among technologists and differences in the time required to perform one exam compared to another" (Goldsmith 2005).

Relative Value Systems

Medicare Physician Fee Schedule

The Medicare program researched RVUs and made them the basis of the Medicare fee schedule starting in 1992. The fee schedule is based on the resource-based relative value scale, or RBRVS. In this Medicare system, the RVU values are weighted geographically using a geographic practice cost index, or GPCI, and then multiplied by a national conversion factor (dollar value) to determine the Medicare-approved amount for each procedure code.

The CMS RVU values are published quarterly and available in the PFS Relative Value Files section of the CMS website (see online appendix G). CMS in the PFS Relative Value Files section of the site. Both current and historical values are available for download.

The RBRVS values are used to determine the approved amount for a Medicare payment. The general formula for calculating Medicare payment amounts for 2013 is expressed as:

[(wRVU × wGPCI) + (peRVU × peGPCI) + (mRVU × mGPCI)] × CF = $

Where:

wRVU = Work RVU component

peRVU = Practice expense RVU component

mRVU = Malpractice expense RVU component

CF = Conversion factor ($34.0230 for 2013)

$ = Medicare-approved amount

Using this formula, the approved amount for CPT code 99213 in Chicago, IL, for 2013 is calculated as:

[(wRVU × wGPCI) + (peRVU × peGPCI) + (mRVU × mGPCI)] × CF = $

[(.97 × 1.030) + (1.10 × 1.051) + (0.07 × 2.077)] × CF = $

[0.9991 + 1.1561 + 0.1454] × CF = $

2.3006 × 34.0230 = $78.31

Relative Values for Physicians (RVPs)

It should be noted that Medicare did not develop the RVU concept. Prior to implementation of the RBRVS by CMS, McGraw-Hill developed and published *Relative Values for Physicians (RVP)*, now published by Optum. RVPs are different from the CMS value system and should not be confused with the CMS version. RVP does not have the subunit values, such as the physician work RVU, that are found in the CMS version.

Note that RVP does have values for some services where Medicare does not, such as laboratory services, causing the temptation to use parts of the value scales interchangeably. However, care should be taken to not mix values between the systems, as they were developed using very different methodologies. Still, the RVP can provide meaningful data. Some analysts calculate the value of physician services using both RVPs and RVUs to provide a complete set of data for comparison, being careful to clearly mark the source of each set of values.

RVU Analysis

RVU data aggregation can be done by physician, by clinic, by specialty, or by service line. For example, physician practices can be compared based on the raw number of encounters, patients, and procedures. However, total RVUs, RVUs per patient, and RVUs per procedure provide additional data that are more descriptive, as displayed in table 8.8. Table 8.8 shows the physician production by CPT range for procedures, encounters, and wRVUs for Doctor #1 of My Town Family Practice, SC.

Table 8.8 Procedures, encounters, and wRVUs by CPT range

Doctor # 1 My Town Family Practice, SC July 20XX						
CPT Range	No. of Proc	%	No. of Encounters	%	wRVU	%
E/M codes (99200–99499)	698	31.0%	449	39.5%	1,035.06	47.62%
Surgery (10000–69999)	146	6.5%	71	6.2%	140.62	6.47%
Radiology (70000–79999)	134	6.0%	74	6.5%	127.98	5.89%
Lab and Path (80000–89999)	392	17.4%	333	29.2%	20.24	.93%
Medicine (90000–99199)	878	39.1%	212	18.6%	849.49	39.09%
Total	2,248	100%	1,139	100%	2,173.39	100%

Physician Productivity

The physician work RVU (wRVU) is commonly used to track physician productivity in healthcare today. It provides a comparative value for work across all specialties. It should be noted, however, that the wRVU component is only a measure of the physician's clinical work, not a measure of the physician's overall work on behalf of the physician practice or the hospital. Research work, management duties, and teaching physician responsibilities should be tracked using other methods.

To accurately perform wRVU analysis, analysts should determine and use the full-time equivalent (FTE) associated with the clinical work. This is called the clinical FTE (cFTE) and should be calculated for all providers. For example, a physician who works four eight-hour days a week in a clinic, does no hospital rounds, and does not take call would have a cFTE of 32 hours divided by 40 hours, or 0.80 (Glass 2008).

Table 8.9 shows a sample productivity report with physicians working a variety of different cFTEs. Note that Dr. 4 works 0.4 cFTE but is producing more wRVUs than the average of the group during this time period. Without using cFTE to equalize the data, Dr. 4 would look like an underperformer.

When analyzing RVUs, averages and ratios are commonly used. In table 8.9, RVUs are displayed as a ratio with encounters and procedures, and the group ratio is shown as an average.

Table 8.9 Physician productivity

Physician Productivity July 20XX My Town Family Practice, SC					
	Dr. 1	Dr. 2	Dr. 3	Dr. 4	Total
wRVUs	2173.39	1383.54	1201.23	732.41	5490.57
Encounters	1,139	608	672	342	2761.00
Procedures	2,248	1,278	1,183	708	5417.00
cFTE status	1	0.8	0.8	0.4	3
Average					
Procedures/ encounters	1.97	2.10	1.76	2.07	1.98
wRVUs/encounters	1.91	2.28	1.79	2.14	2.03
wRVUs/procedures	0.97	1.08	1.02	1.03	1.02
wRVUs/cFTE	2173	1729	1502	1831	1809
Encounters/cFTE	1139	760	840	855	899
Procedures/cFTE	2248	1598	1479	1770	1774

Service Line Analysis

Mindy Goldsmith, PhD, describes the process of evaluating the Radiology Department of a general hospital using RVUs in "Apple to Apples—RVU Analysis in Radiology." This article points out the power of analysis by RVUs for any service where CPT codes, and therefore RVU values, are assigned. The author suggests calculating total RVUs by exam type, average RVUs per day, and average RVUs per FTE in the department. The author also suggests calculating the cost per RVU for the department and for individual modalities and the cost per RVU for each type of expense such as supplies, equipment maintenance, technologist salaries, and administrative overhead (clerks, transcriptionists, and management staff) (Goldsmith 2005).

Average Cost per RVU

Physician practices can evaluate contracts that pay by a set dollar amount per RVU if they know the practice's average cost per RVU. Contracts that pay a higher dollar value per RVU than the average cost per RVU have the greatest chance at creating profitability for the practice. Therefore, the average cost per RVU is also referred to as the break-even conversion factor (BECF).

Calculating the Average Cost per RVU

To calculate the average cost per RVU, follow these steps:

List all CPT codes used by the practice in a spreadsheet, along with the associated RVU components from CMS for physician work, practice expense, and malpractice expense. Weight each of these components by the appropriate GPCI for the location of the practice and total the RVU components for each code.

List the frequency that each CPT code was used by the practice within the same time period and multiply the frequency by the total weighted RVU for each code. (Be sure the frequencies are weighted for modifier use, such as modifier –50 = 150 percent of the base RVU, modifier –51 = 50 percent of the base RVU, modifiers –80, –81, and –82 = 16 percent of the base RVU.) Total the RVUs produced for the period.

Obtain the amount of the total expenses for the same time period from the statement of revenue and expenses. Divide the total expenses by total RVUs to determine the average cost per RVU.

Calculate the cost associated with any CPT code by multiplying the average cost per RVU by the relative weight for that CPT code.

Other Data Calculations Using RVUs

In addition to the average cost per RVU, other measures can be compared to RVUs. Three common comparisons are physician compensation per wRVU, malpractice expense per mRVU, and overhead (practice expense) per peRVU.

Physician Compensation per wRVU

To determine how much a practice pays the provider staff, use the formula of:

$$Cost\,per\,wRVU = \frac{Total\,Provider\,Compensation\,Expenses}{Total\,wRVU}$$

Practices can define the provider compensation expenses in any way that they choose, being sure to maintain consistency from year to year. Some practices include all expenses that can be directly allocated to the physician in this calculation, while others use the salary, employee payroll tax, basic insurance costs, and retirement plan costs as the only expenses. Nonphysician practitioners can be combined into these calculations or calculated separately, based on practice preference.

Malpractice Expense per mRVU

This calculation determines the cost of malpractice insurance coverage per mRVU that is produced. To calculate the cost per mRVU, use the formula of:

$$Cost\,per\,wRVU = \frac{Total\,Provider\,Malpractice\,Expenses}{Total\,wRVU}$$

The practice should use the same method here for nonphysician practitioners that was used for physician compensation, either combined into the total or calculated separately.

Overhead (Practice Expense) per peRVU

The most difficult part of determining the overhead per peRVU is to determine which expenses go into the overhead category. The easiest way to determine this is to calculate the physician compensation and malpractice ratios first. All of the other practice expenses not accounted for in those two ratios then belong in the overhead per peRVU ratio. If the expense cannot be directly related to physician compensation or to malpractice premium expense, include it in the overhead calculation. To calculate the cost per peRVU, use the formula of:

$$Cost\,per\,peRVU = \frac{Total\,Provider\,Overhead\,Expenses}{Total\,peRVU}$$

Break-Even Conversion Factor (BECF)

The break-even conversion factor (BECF) can be calculated from a grouping of fees and used to help negotiate payment contracts. The average cost per RVU formula (total expenses divided by total RVUs equals cost per RVU) can be modified to show the conversion factor used to create a fee schedule. This formula would be:

$$BECF = \frac{Total\,Practice\,Expenses}{Total\,RVUs}$$

This calculated conversion factor can then be compared to the current Medicare conversion factor and the conversion factor used to establish the fees for the practice. The difference between the practice's cost per RVU and the conversion factor used to create the payer's fee schedule is the potential profit to be made from the services provided to that payer.

 Review Questions

1. An analyst wishes to use the CMI for a set of MS-DRGs to determine if a documentation improvement program is having an impact. Use the MS-DRG volumes and weights in the table below to calculate the CMI for the three MS-DRGs.

MS-DRG	Description	Weight	Volume
034	CAROTID ARTERY STENT PROCEDURE W MCC	3.6918	100
035	CAROTID ARTERY STENT PROCEDURE W CC	2.1965	52
036	CAROTID ARTERY STENT PROCEDURE W/O CC/MCC	1.6610	36

   a. 2.3234
   b. 2.8893
   c. 2.5164
   d. 3.6918

2. An increasing CMI is indicative of which trend?
   a. Increasing patient resource intensity
   b. Decreasing payment per case
   c. Increasing proportion of surgical patients
   d. Increasing cost of living

3. Which of the following influence CMI?
   a. Length of stay in special care units
   b. Coding and documentation
   c. Number of lab tests ordered per stay
   d. Total charges

4. APR-DRGs are an extension of the DRG system that include:
   a. Indicators for mortality risk and severity
   b. Indicators for mortality risk only
   c. Inclusion of pediatric DRGs
   d. Indicators for patient severity

5. Bell curve analysis may be used to determine if:
   a. A provider is missing charges
   b. Evaluation and management level criteria are reasonable
   c. OCE errors will be encountered
   d. Productivity standards are met

6. Which of the following is not a difference between APC and MS-DRGs?
   a. APC weights are based on resource intensity and MS-DRG weights are not
   b. MS-DRG weights are standardized to 1.0 and APC weights are not
   c. A claim may have more than one APC, but only one MS-DRG
   d. MS-DRGs are used to determine Medicare payments and APCs are not

7. Relative Value Units are:
   a. Weights assigned to APC codes to measure resource intensity
   b. Weights assigned to DRG codes to measure resource intensity
   c. Weights assigned to CPT codes to measure resource intensity
   d. Weights assigned to physicians to measure productivity

8. If the total fees paid to a physician practice equal $105,000 and the total RVUs during that same time period was 3,000 units. What is the BECF?
   a. $34.03
   b. $35.00
   c. $39.23
   d. $30.00

9. Which of the following metrics may be used to measure physician productivity?
   a. Total RVUs
   b. Work RVUs (wRVU)
   c. Practice Expense RVUs (peRVU)
   d. Malpractice expense RVUs (mRVU)

10. What are the components of the Medicare RVUs?
    a. Work, practice expense, conversion factor
    b. Work, practice expense, malpractice expense
    c. Work and malpractice expense
    d. Practice expense, overhead expense, malpractice expense

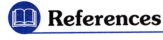 References

Bryant, G. 2008 (May 15). AHIMA Audio Seminar: Managing the CMI Under MS-DRGs.

Casto, A. and E. Forrestal. 2012. *Principles of Healthcare Reimbursement*, 4th ed. Chicago: AHIMA.

Centers for Medicare and Medicaid Services. (2012). *Specifications Manual for National Hospital Inpatient Quality Measures Version 4.2a*. Baltimore: CMS.

CMS. (2012, October). *Hospital-Acquired Conditions (HAC) in Acute Inpatient Prospective Payment System (IPPS) Hospitals. Medicare Learning Network*. Baltimore: Department of Health and Human Services.

Goldsmith, M. 2005. Apple to apples—RVU analysis in radiology. *Radiology Today* 6(11):14.

Hanna, J. 2002. Constructing a coding compliance plan. *Journal of AHIMA* 73(7): 48–56.

Wilson, D. and R. Dunn. 2009. *Benchmarking to Improve Coding Accuracy and Productivity*. Chicago: AHIMA.

Wozniak, L. 2002. Monitoring and evaluating your hospital's inpatient case mix. *AHIMA's 74th National Convention and Exhibit Proceedings*.

Benchmarking and Analyzing Externally Reported Data

In today's healthcare environment, healthcare organizations provide data voluntarily and upon mandate to outside organizations. These organizations, both public and private, evaluate the data in comparison to their criteria and report the results of the comparison to purchasers of the data or to the public.

When it comes to studying a healthcare organization's published results, data analysts play a role, both in determining reasonability and for performance improvement. This chapter discusses benchmarking, a commonly used method for collecting and comparing data, as well as some of the organizations that collect and report data.

The Benchmarking Process

Benchmarking is a management tool that drives performance and quality improvement by allowing comparison of performance to an established standard (Glass 2008). The American Productivity and Quality Center (APQC) describes benchmarking as "the process of improving performance by continuously identifying, understanding and adapting outstanding practices and processes found inside and outside the organization" (APQC 1999).

There are two types of benchmarking: internal and external. **Internal benchmarking** is performed by comparing an organization's performance over time. In order to assess their competitive position, providers must perform **external benchmarking**. For clinical projects, external sources of clinical benchmarking data must be identified. Medicare claims may be purchased from Centers for Medicare and Medicaid Services (CMS) under the Freedom of Information Act. All payer claims data are more difficult to obtain.

When integrating internal and external clinical data, the analyst must be careful that the time frames are comparable. For instance, a comparison of outpatient claims from 2006 summarized by the ambulatory payment classification (APC) to internal outpatient claims from 2009 may or may not be valid. For some APCs, the code assignments may have changed, compromising the validity of the comparison.

This chapter will review the process of benchmarking and the sources for external data for quality and efficiency benchmarking.

The Benefits of Benchmarking

Benchmarking can benefit an organization by helping to identify weak areas and the potential for improvement. It can also confirm the belief that there is a need for improvement and challenge organizational complacency with the status quo (SM Thacker 2000). Further, it can demonstrate that levels of performance that were once thought acceptable may no longer be seen that way by a customer or the industry.

In healthcare, facilities use benchmarking as part of their quality improvement culture. For example, Womack and Jones presented the **lean thinking model** to maximize value and minimize waste, while **Six Sigma** was created to identify and remove the cause of errors (Womack and Jones 2003).

Steps in the Benchmarking Process

The amount and complexity of benchmarking activities performed within an organization are determined by the amount of comparative data and other resources available for the work. The benchmarking process for data analysis involves the following steps:

1. Identify the issue to benchmark
2. Locate internal data related to the issue
3. Analyze internal data
4. Identify external data available for benchmarking
5. Collect public domain data or purchase data, if appropriate
6. Compare internal and external data
7. Determine whether a performance gap exists
8. Communicate benchmarking findings
9. Establish performance-level targets and action plans for achievement
10. Implement plans; monitor and communicate progress
11. Recalibrate benchmarks as necessary
12. Repeat the process

Dashboard Reports and Scorecards

A **dashboard report** is a method of presenting data about the key performance indicators for an organization; it functions in a manner similar to the dashboard of a car. The data included on the dashboard provide valuable information that is in an easily readable format and can be used as a guide for making management decisions. Dashboards are oftentimes the method used to communicate findings of the benchmarking process and ongoing performance.

Dashboards should include a combination of per-unit quantitative indicators which provide a better picture of overall performance than any one indicator. Kathryn Glass, an industry expert in analyzing physician data, recommends including indicators in the categories of clinical, operational, and financial data (Glass 2008).

Dashboard reports are easily created in Microsoft Excel. Add-on programs are available for the Microsoft Excel program, and Microsoft Office website has basic templates available for creating dashboard reports. Appendix B includes a demonstration of the analytic capabilities found in Excel. However, specialized programs that involve print-ready graphics are also available for creating dashboards.

Figure 9.1 is a sample dashboard for a typical physician practice and is provided as part of the online resources as Physician_Dashboard.xls.

Figure 9.1   **Physician dashboard**

Dashboard for William Michaels, MD, Hospitalist
July 31, 20XX

	Michaels	Other Hospitalists	Hospitalist Group
wRVUs	953.87	3544.05	4497.91
Procedures	591	1914	2505
cFTE Status	1	3	4
wRVUs/Procedure	1.61	1.85	1.80
wRVUs/cFTE	954	1181	1124
Procedures/cFTE	591	638	626
Procedure Break-out			
Surgery	25	121	146
Medicine	23	109	132
E&M	543	1684	2227
Total	591	1914	2505

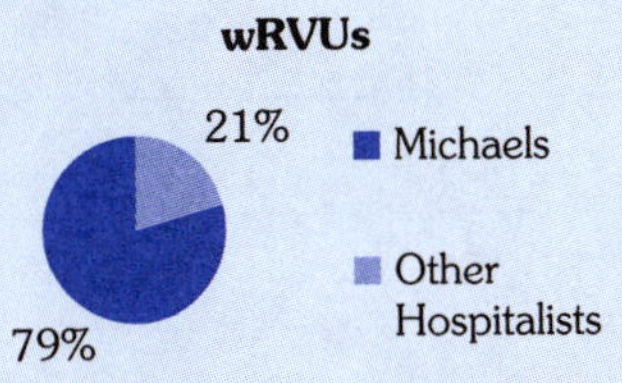

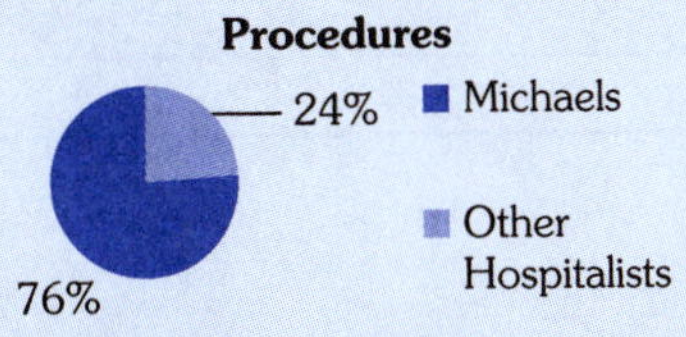

(continued)

Figure 9.1 Physician dashboard (*continued*)

Dashboard for William Michaels, MD, Hospitalist
July 31, 20XX

Initial Hospital Visits			MGMA Benchmark	
99221	63	50%	35%	
99222	23	18%	23%	
99223	39	31%	42%	
	125	100%	100%	
Subsequent Hosp Visits			MGMA Benchmark	
99231	116	35%	31%	
99232	153	46%	55%	
99233	62	19%	14%	
	331	100%	100%	
Hospital Consultations			MGMA Benchmark	
99251	2	3%	6%	
99252	4	6%	12%	
99253	23	33%	27%	
99254	23	33%	35%	
99255	18	26%	20%	
	70	100%	100%	

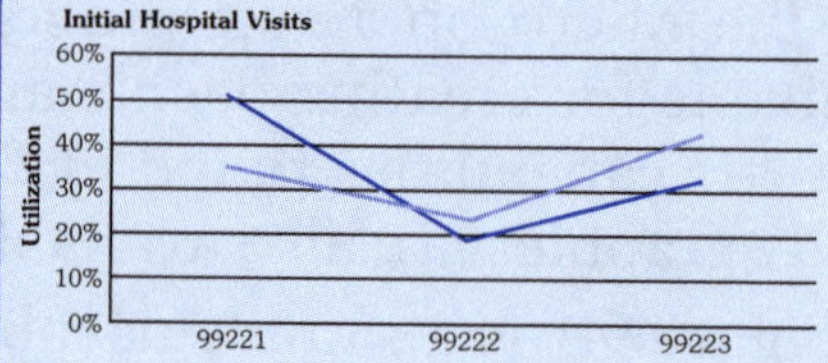

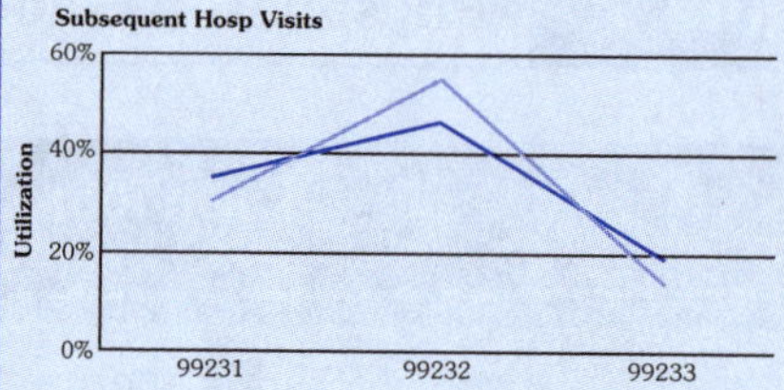

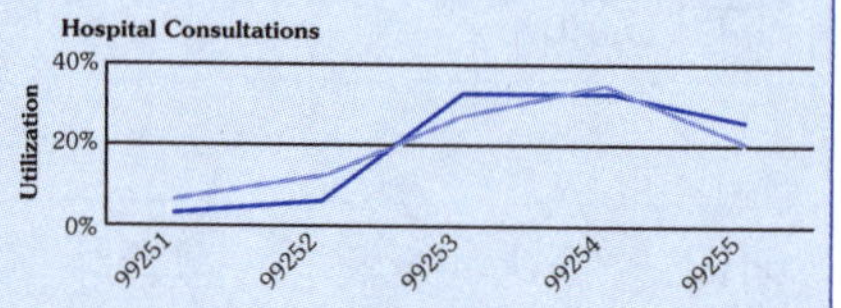

Figure 9.2 is a sample dashboard report for a typical hospital.

Some dashboards are more graphic than others. For example, the Agency for Healthcare Research and Quality (AHRQ) uses dashboards on its website to display the degree of performance for each state for several categories of quality indicators. The AHRQ dashboards are available on their website by clicking on the "State Selection Map" link and choosing a particular state (see online appendix G). The state-specific data is displayed using meter graphs and provides immediate information on the state's performance in several different areas. The meter for overall health quality is shown

Figure 9.2 **Hospital dashboard**

System Dashboard (November, 20xx)				
	Baseline	**Target**	**Previous Result**	**Current Result**
Clinical Performance				
Clinical Indicator #1	93%	>98%	96% ▸	97% ▸
Clinical Indicator #2	86%	>92%	92% ■	93% ■
Clinical Indicator #3	76%	>82%	81% ▸	82% ■
Clinical Indicator #4	82%	>79%	88% ■	97% ■
Clinical Indicator #5	23%	<24%	22% ■	22% ■
Clinical Indicator #6	47%	>47%	49% ■	49% ■
Patient Safety				
Safety Indicator #1	1.18	<0.90	1.14 ▸	1.1 ▸
Safety Indicator #2	1.66	<0.91	1.75 ◂	1.74 ◂
Safety Indicator #3	1.49	<0.68	1.19 ▸	1.18 ▸
Safety Indicator #4	0.65	<0.72	0.62 ■	0.61 ■
Safety Indicator #5	1%	>60%	20% ▸	19% ▸
Safety Indicator #6	33%	>70%	36% ▸	37% ▸
System Scaled Score	**80**	**100 (0-100)**		**92**

◂ Result worse than baseline
▸ Result better than baseline, but worse than target
■ Result meets or exceeds target

Last updated on 12/5/12

in figure 9.3. The dashboard includes measures of performance segmented by three categories:

1. Types of care
   a. Preventive measures
   b. Acute care measures
   c. Chronic care measures

2. Settings of care
   a. Hospital care measures

Figure 9.3 **AHRQ dashboard example**

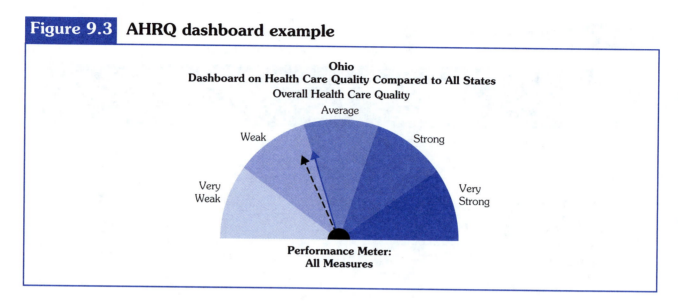

b. Ambulatory care measures
c. Home health care measures

3. Care by clinical area

   a. Cancer measures
   b. Diabetes measures
   c. Heart disease measures
   d. Maternal and child health measures
   e. Respiratory diseases measures

The dashed line on the meter represents the state's baseline value and the solid line represents the most recent value.

Report Card Data and Quality Reporting

Healthcare organizations are asked to report data for quality measurement purposes. A **quality measure** is a mechanism that enables the user to quantify the quality of a selected aspect of care by comparing it to a criterion. For example, a clinical performance measure is a mechanism for assessing the degree to which a provider competently and safely delivers clinical services that are appropriate for the patient in the optimal time period. A quality measure converts medical information from patient records into a rate or percentage that allows facilities to assess their performance (Hazelwood 2008). Note that organizations seeking to improve their performance benchmark their data against the data of organizations that are performing at the highest levels.

Government entities (CMS, AHRQ) and private organizations concerned about quality (The Joint Commission, the National Committee for Quality Assurance) request data for quality measurement. Many of these requests are voluntary; however, some may be mandatory for participation in particular payment plans. In addition, CMS announced in the rules for both the inpatient prospective payment system (IPPS) and outpatient prospective payment system (OPPS) that failure to report quality measure data will result in a 2 percent reduction from the market basket update to the conversion factor for the associated facilities. As Medicare payment evolves from a pay for reporting to a true value-based pay for performance system, the measurement of quality indicators will be increasingly important.

In chapter 3 we discussed how small-scale databases may be built specifically for quality reporting. An example would be that a data analyst or programmer designs and populates a database for the acute myocardial infarction indicators with those patients who were coded and grouped into MS-DRG 282, Acute myocardial infarction, discharged alive without complication or comorbidity (CC) or major complication or comorbidity (MCC). This population forms the denominator for the calculation of the indicator. Following this, the quality reviewer would evaluate the documentation using each set of criteria that relates to this diagnosis, such as the aspirin on arrival indicator (Acute myocardial infarction patients without aspirin contraindication who received aspirin within 24 hours before or after hospital arrival). The reviewer would note if aspirin was given according to the timeframes listed in the indicator. The reviewer would also note if the patient had a contraindication to aspirin such as an allergy, Coumadin as a prearrival medication, or active bleeding. In the case of a contraindication, the case would be marked to be excluded from the denominator because it did not meet the criteria.

After the data has been reported, the data analyst may be asked to determine how the facility's data compare to that of other facilities in the city, state, region, or nation. This is done by accessing public data from the organization that requested the data.

The following is a description of some of the public and private organizations involved in quality reporting and the data they collect and display. This list is not intended to be exhaustive.

Hospital Compare

Hospital Compare reports on 94 measures of hospital quality of care for heart attack, heart failure, pneumonia, and the prevention of surgical infections. The data available at Hospital Compare is reported by hospitals to meet the requirements of the Medicare Value Based Purchasing program. Providers that report the indicators receive the full annual payment update for IPPS and OPPS. CMS will eventually move to reporting based on the demonstrated improvement in the indicators. A complete set of indicators can be found on their website (see appendix G).

- Structural Measures (6 measures)
- Timely and Effective Care (Process of Care Measures)
  - Heart Attack (Acute myocardial infarction (AMI)) (8)
  - Heart Failure (3)
  - Pneumonia (2)
  - Surgery (Surgical Care Improvement Project) (9)
  - Emergency Department Care (7)

○ Preventive Care (2)

○ Children's Asthma Care (2)

● Readmissions, Complications, and Deaths (Outcome of Care Measures)
  ○ 30-day death (mortality) rates and 30-day readmission rates (6)
  ○ Serious complications—AHRQ Patient Safety Indicators (PSIs) (19)
  ○ Hospital-acquired conditions (8)
  ○ Healthcare-associated infections (4)

● Use of Medical Imaging (Outpatient Imaging Efficiency Measures) (6)
● Survey of Patients' Hospital Experiences (HCAHPS (Hospital Consumer Assessment of Healthcare Providers and Systems)) (10)
● Number of Medicare patients (1)
● Spending per hospital patient with Medicare (1)

[CMS, n.d.]

Figure 9.4 displays the comparison of three Chicago-area hospitals for the Antibiotics at the Right Time indicator.

The Leapfrog Group

The Leapfrog organization is a consortium of large companies and private and public healthcare purchasers. Leapfrog's mission, according to their website, is triggering giant leaps forward in the safety, quality, and affordability of healthcare by supporting healthcare decisions made by those who use and pay for healthcare as well as promoting high-value healthcare through incentives and rewards.

Figure 9.4   Antibiotic within one hour before surgery

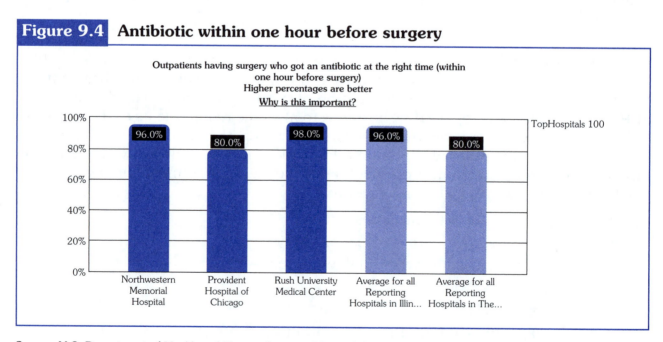

Source: U.S. Department of Health and Human Services, Hospital Compare Data.

The Leapfrog Group collects and distributes data through the Leapfrog Hospital Survey. Any hospital is eligible to report data. Once the data are compared to Leapfrog Group criteria, they are reported at the Leapfrog Group website in the form of a scorecard (see online appendix G). The scorecard reports on six vital areas for hospitals:

- Prevention of medication errors
- Appropriate ICU staffing with professionals specially trained in critical care
- Steps to avoid harm
- Reduction of pressure ulcers
- Reduction of in-hospital injuries
- Managing serious errors

Figure 9.5 shows a Leapfrog Scorecard for several southern Wisconsin hospitals on the subject of aortic valve replacement surgery.

Bridges to Excellence

Bridges to Excellence is a not-for-profit organization developed by employers, physicians, healthcare services, researchers, and other industry experts. Its mission is to help the best clinicians build their practices, help patients get healthier, help insurers and employers manage costs better, by defining critical indicators (the ones that can most impact quality and financial performance), measuring and reporting on them, and recognizing high performers with incentives. Bridges to Excellence is a pay-for-performance program with a standard data exchange platform and performance measurements, both of which can be implemented through a variety of different models such as state governments, health plans, and employers.

HealthGrades

HealthGrades is a healthcare rating organization. Its website describes its rating system as being based on the most current three-year data set available from CMS and several states that participate. HealthGrades uses statistical techniques to process and risk-adjust patient-level data into easily understandable, objective report card ratings on providers.

Basic data on 31 procedures or diagnoses are available for hospitals, sorted by state and geographic area. More specialized information may be purchased for hospitals, physicians, and nursing homes.

HealthGrades publishes several documents that describe the methodology used in rating hospitals. The documents are found under the HealthGrades for Business section of their Web site by mousing over "Hospital Solutions" and clicking on "Clinical Excellence Research and Consulting." The *Hospital Report Cards™ Mortality and Complications Outcomes 2013 Methodology* describes how the service-area ratings (number of stars) are assigned (see online appendix G). The methodology also gives a general discussion of the procedures or diagnoses that are included in each group. This methodology white paper contains an appendix that details the inclusions and exclusions from each category.

Figure 9.5	**Leapfrog Group hospital quality ratings for aortic valve replacement**

HealthGrades' Methods of Analysis

Example 1:

A hospital receives one star (out of five) for postoperative anemia subsequent to total joint replacements and initiates an investigation into the low-star rating. The action plan is to review the data associated with these procedures and look for obvious issues. The data analyst runs claim histories on all total joint replacement cases and frequency reports of the diagnoses associated with these procedures (chapter 4). The frequency of the postoperative complication code is high, and the data analyst selects these cases for review by the health record auditor. Upon health record review, it is determined that the physicians were documenting "postoperative anemia," and after discussion with the physicians, it is determined that they meant anemia within the postoperative period as an expected complication. They did not mean that these were unexpected postoperative complications. As part of the action plan for follow-up, the coders will review the *AHA Coding Clinic* guidelines for postoperative anemia, while the physicians will receive education on the documentation differences between "anemia" and "postoperative anemia." The physicians will also be queried on any unclear documentation.

Example 2:

A hospital sees that HealthGrades has given it a higher than average death rate for the principal diagnosis of sepsis. (The hospital has a palliative care program and frequently sees patients who are terminally ill.) The data analyst at the hospital is asked to investigate and reviews *Mortality and Complication Based Outcomes 2008*, concentrating on the diagnoses that are included and excluded for the category of sepsis. The analyst studies the frequency of diagnoses associated with the sepsis cases and determines that the

V66.7 encounter for palliative care code is not being assigned by the coders. This code would exclude these cases from the calculation. As part of the action plan for follow-up, the coders will review the documentation required for the assignment of this code, while the physicians will receive education on the documentation of palliative care. The physicians will also be queried on any unclear documentation.

The National Committee for Quality Assurance (NCQA) and the Healthcare Effectiveness Data and Information Set (HEDIS)

The National Committee for Quality Assurance (NCQA) is a private, not-for-profit organization dedicated to assessing and reporting on the quality of healthcare plans as well as improving healthcare quality. It is governed by a board of directors that includes employers, consumer and labor representatives, health plans, quality experts, policy makers, and representatives from organized medicine.

NCQA's mission is to provide information that enables purchasers and consumers of managed healthcare to distinguish among plans based on quality, thereby allowing them to make more informed healthcare purchasing decisions. This encourages plans to compete based on quality and value, rather than on price and provider network. NCQA's efforts are organized around two activities, accreditation and performance measurement, which are complementary strategies for producing information to guide choice.

HEDIS, developed and maintained by NCQA, is used by health plans to collect data about the quality of care and service they provide. It consists of a set of performance measures that evaluate how well health plans perform in key domains: effectiveness of care, access or availability of care, use of services, cost of care, and member satisfaction with the experience of care. HEDIS requires health plans to collect data in a standardized way so that comparisons are fair and valid.

An individual HEDIS measure is made up of the measure name and a description of the care, screening, or test needed. Each measure specifies the criteria for denominator (the eligible population) and numerator inclusion (those who received the care). For example, a measure in the effectiveness of care domain is "comprehensive diabetes care," with a description that reads:

The percentage of members 18–75 years of age with diabetes (type 1 and type 2) who have had each of the following:

- Hemoglobin A1c (HbA1c) testing
- HbA1c poor control (> 9.0%)
- HbA1c control (< 8.0%)
- HbA1c control (< 7.0%)
- LDL-C screening
- LDL-C control (< 100 mg/dL)
- Eye exam (retinal) performed
- Medical attention for nephropathy
- Blood pressure control < 140/90 mm Hg
- Blood pressure control < 130/80 mm Hg

In the previous example, note that while there is a single measure for diabetes, there are 10 indicators within the measure. Generally speaking, a plan may elect to report only one or all indicators for a given measure. Criteria for each indicator include codes to help identify numerator-positive events such as HbA1c tests or eye examinations, which include a retinal evaluation. In each measure, each indicator must be programmed separately.

To determine the exact criteria and collection methodology, the data analyst must reference the complete set of measures and the associated technical specifications for data collection. Some HEDIS measures are reported using only administrative (claims-based) data, whereas others can be reported hybrid via a combination of administrative data and health record data.

During HEDIS data collection, data analysts may do the programming to retrieve data or may work with programming staff that complete this task for them. An important step in this process is for the programmer to have the programming code validated against the specifications prior to formal data analysis. Usually, the programmer will have a peer conduct this validation, which could involve a test run of the data to look at the data's reasonability. An additional step may involve having a formal source code (programming language) review. A healthcare organization may do its own programming for data reporting or may opt to use a software program that is NCQA-certified. For either of these options, the source code reviewer would review the program code against the specifications for each measure being reported to ensure that specification parameters are programmed correctly.

A final validation is also performed, which is called "primary source verification." This step helps ensure that the data found in the output file are also present in the data source files (claims or encounters and enrollment or eligibility) and confirms the programming adheres to measure specifications. A list of numerator-positive cases is run, and a random sample is selected. The list would include data elements used to locate the member (insured) within the information system(s) as well as the date of service that qualified the member for the numerator. The date of service would also be used to confirm that the member met continuous enrollment criteria by checking the member's eligibility spans in the organization's eligibility system. In addition, the numerator event (diagnosis code, procedure code, Type of Bill, or Place of Service) for that date of service must be verified in the claims or encounter system. Primary source verification may not catch any or all programming errors, but is a good practice nevertheless.

Another crucial step is to ensure that the programmer maintains documentation on the procedures used to pull data for any reports that are critical in the organization. A step-by-step document will help ensure the organization's ability to replicate important reports. The programmer should also be mindful to track the version of the programming code (including dates the code was revised) either within the program code itself or within the step-by-step document.

In order to publicly report their rates, health plans must arrange to have their HEDIS results verified by a licensed organization (LO) or an independent auditor who is a certified HEDIS compliance auditor (CHCA) under the supervision of an LO. Individuals with experience in data analysis often are employed by an LO in the role of auditor.

Measures reported via hybrid are subject to an accuracy overread by the auditor or LO to ensure that health record data were collected according to specifications. In addition to auditing data collection methods set up by the data analyst, the auditor will review information systems, data processing, system compliance with measure specifications, and—finally—the rates generated by the plan's programming. The rates are reviewed for reasonability and compared to national benchmarks as well as to previous year's rates in order to identify potential issues. This entire process can take over two years to accomplish.

Health plans are not the only ones who find HEDIS valuable. Employers and consumers use HEDIS rates to evaluate health plan performance across specific domains to determine whether or not they wish to contract with the plans for healthcare service delivery. Plans who achieve NCQA Accreditation can earn excellent status by having HEDIS rates in the highest range of national and regional performance. In addition, plans that offer a Medicaid product may be mandated by the state to participate in HEDIS reporting activities, and rates may be used to evaluate the plan's degree of compliance with state standards.

✔ Review Questions

1. What is the benefit of benchmarking?
   a. Identify areas for improvement
   b. Demonstrate level of performance
   c. Isolate the cause of errors
   d. All of the above

2. What is the first step in a benchmarking project?
   a. Collect comparative data
   b. Collect internal data
   c. Analyze data
   d. Identify the issue to be benchmarked

3. Dashboards are:
   a. A graphical display of performance on key metrics
   b. A statistical inference tool
   c. A data collection tool
   d. Used to determine root cause of quality issues

4. AHRQ is the:
   a. Agency for Healthcare Resource and Quality
   b. Agency for Healthcare Reference and Quantity
   c. Agency for Hospital Revenue and Quality
   d. Agency for Healthcare Research and Quality

5. Which of these settings is not measured as part of the AHRQ quality dashboards?
   a. Hospitals
   b. Ambulatory care
   c. Physician care
   d. Home health care

6. How are hospital compare measures used by CMS?
   a. Hospitals that score better than average receive bonus payments
   b. Hospitals that report all measures receive the full payment update
   c. Hospitals that perform poorly must pay a penalty
   d. Hospital payment is not impacted by hospital compare indicators

7. Which of the following quality measurement groups was created by private healthcare purchasers?
   a. AHRQ
   b. HEDIS
   c. Leagfrog Group
   d. Hospital Compare

8. Which of the following quality measurement group measures the performance of managed care organizations?
   a. AHRQ
   b. HEDIS
   c. Leagfrog Group
   d. Hospital Compare

9. Which of the following is a good source of benchmark data for hospitals?
   a. USA Today
   b. HEDIS
   c. NCQA
   d. Hospital Compare

10. Which of the following quality measurement group measures physician quality?
   a. HEDIS
   b. Hospital Compare
   c. Healthgrades
   d. AHRQ

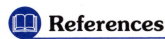

References

American Productivity & Quality Center (APQC). 1999. Benchmarking: Leveraging Best-Practice Strategies, an APQC White Paper for Senior Management Based on the Internationally Acclaimed Study. Organizing and Managing Benchmarking. http://www .isixsigma.com/offsite.asp?A=Fr&Url=http://www.apqc.org/portal/apqc/ksn?paf_gear_ id=contentgearhome&paf_dm=full&pageselect=include&docid=112421

Centers for Medicare and Medicaid Services. (n.d.). Hospital Compare. http://www.medicare. gov/hospitalcompare/

Glass, K. 2008. *RVUs: Applications for Medical Practice Success*, 2nd ed. Englewood: Medical Group Management Association.

Hazelwood, A. 2008. AHIMA Distance Education Course: Data Reporting for Quality Initiatives. http://www.ahima.org

HealthGrades. 2008. Methodology White Paper. http://www.healthgrades.com/media/DMS/ pdf/HospitalReportCardsMortalityComplications2009.pdf

SM Thacker & Associates. 2000. An introduction to benchmarking. http://www.smthacker .co.uk/introduction_to_benchmarking.htm

Womack, J.P. and D.T. Jones. 2003. *Lean Thinking: Banish Waste and Create Wealth in Your Corporation*, revised and updated. New York: Simon & Schuster Adult Publishing Group.

Appendix A: Understanding Databases

(Adapted from: White, S. 2013. Understanding databases. Chapter 4 in *Introduction to Healthcare Informatics*. Chicago: AHIMA.)

Healthcare is a data-rich business. On the business side of healthcare, claims are generated and submitted for payment. Payment transactions are then sent back to the provider. On the clinical side of healthcare, countless diagnostic tests are performed and the results of those tests are provided back to practitioners and providers. The introduction of the electronic health record (EHR) and sophisticated EHR systems increased the amount of data available in the healthcare setting exponentially. The Centers for Medicare and Medicaid Services' (CMS) meaningful use criteria, value-based purchasing programs, and the formation of Accountable Care Organizations (ACOs) and other payment reform policies are driving the need for providers to use the data produced during the delivery of care to help improve the efficiency and effectiveness of the healthcare system. If these goals are to be met, then the data must be organized in a way that allows analysis and reports to be produced accurately and in real time. Databases give structure to the raw data and facilitate the manipulation of data to achieve these goals.

Database Terminology

Prior to studying the various types of databases and database management systems (DBMSs), it is important to have a common set of terminology to describe the various components of a database. Databases may be envisioned as a collection of data tables. The most common form of a data table found in practice is a tab or worksheet within a spreadsheet.

Table A.1 Patients and their appointments

Patient_ID	Provider_ID	Appointment_Date	Appointment_Time
ABD239	SMI123	1/23/2012	9:00 a.m.
DIR235	SMI123	1/23/2012	9:30 a.m.
JKF764	SMI123	1/23/2012	10:00 a.m.

Data tables include records or rows, and fields or columns. For example, table A.1 represents a table of patients and their associated appointments. The fields in this table represent data elements describing attributes of the appointment (provider, date, and time). A collection of fields that are related are placed in the same record. The records in this table represent the data describing the patient's appointment. Records in a data table may represent patient demographic information, attributes of a service provided to a patient, or even a diagnostic or procedural code (such as ICD-9) and its definition.

Sets of records include a common set of fields and are related to the same business purpose or focuses are collected together into a data table. There are common data tables found in healthcare:

- Patient demographics
- Physician specialty and licensure
- Charge description master (CDM)
- Patient services

A collection of data tables is called a database. Databases can have a variety of structures and may be created and maintained using a DBMS. A DBMS provides a method for adding or deleting data and also supports methods to extract data for reporting.

Types of Databases

To decide on the type of database that is most appropriate to store data, the user must answer some key questions:

- How many records will the database contain (currently and in the foreseeable future)?
- How do the variables relate to each other?
- What database tools are available for use?
- How will the data be pulled or queried from the database?

The answers to these questions will drive the database type. There typically is not a right or wrong answer in database design. If the database is robust enough to hold all of the information required and extracting information is straightforward, then it should be considered a good quality design. The two most common types of databases used in practice are flat files, or data tables, and relational databases.

Flat Files

If the data structure is relatively simple, then a flat file or spreadsheet may be the right type of database. For instance, if a practice manager wished to track the number of records coded by each employee, then the flat file displayed in table A.2 is sufficient.

Table A.2 Flat file example

Employee	Monday	Tuesday	Wednesday	Thursday	Friday	Weekly Total
Anne	4	9	6	6	5	30
Nicholas	6	10	7	3	6	32
Zach	4	7	9	8	4	32

This structure allows the manager to see who is the most or least productive and may be expanded by adding additional columns to track more days. A series of flat files or individual spreadsheets may be used to track other information about the employees, such as credentials or continuing education (CEU) credits. If the number of additional attributes is small, then they may be added to the records displayed in table A.2. If there is a large number of additional attributes, they may be stored in a second flat file.

Flat file databases may be stored in a number of formats. Traditional spreadsheet tabs, such as those found in Microsoft Excel, are the most common format found in business applications. Flat files may also be stored in text files as columns of data or with the fields delimited by a character. Table A.3 shows an example of column-delimited data and table A.4 shows the same data stored in a comma-delimited or comma-separated value (CSV) file. Column-delimited data must be accompanied by documentation that lists the order and position of the variables so that the data may be interpreted properly. CSV files may include the variable names in the first row. If not, then they too require documentation to identify the variables in each position.

Table A.3 Column-delimited data

Employee	Monday	Tuesday	Wednesday	Thursday	Friday	Weekly Total
Anne	4	9	6	6	5	30
Nicholas	6	10	7	3	6	32
Zach	4	7	9	8	4	32

Table A.4 Comma-separated values

Employee, Monday, Tuesday, Wednesday, Thursday, Friday, Weekly Total
Anne,4,9,6,6,5,30 Nicholas,6,10,7,3,6,32 Zach,4,7,9,8,4,32

Flat data tables have an intuitive two-dimensional format of rows and columns. The number of rows and columns is limited only by the software tool used to store and analyze the data. If a spreadsheet program is used to store the data, then formulas may be imbedded into the table structure and are stored as part of the data table. A flat data table may be sorted or filtered to select particular values of the variables.

The primary limitation of storing data in flat tables is that the design does not allow relationships between variables in separate tables. This limits the ability to cross check values for data integrity to those variables stored in the same table. For instance, if the CDM includes Current Procedural Terminology (CPT) codes, the validation of the CPT code could only be accomplished by relating the CDM in one table to the CPT code table. The second limitation is that the same data element may need to be stored in multiple tables to allow for useful reporting. Data redundancy is not a good practice in database design and can cause serious data integrity issues when a variable is updated in one table, but not the others in which it is stored. If the tables used to store the various data elements need to be combined or must be validated against each other to ensure data integrity, then a relational database is a better choice.

Relational Databases

Relational databases were first conceptualized by Edgar F. Codd. Codd proposed that data should be stored in a way that allowed users to query and analyze data without having to restructure it (Codd 1970, 377). As an example, suppose a data analyst wished to create a report of the number of patients served by zip code and clinical department. The data reside in two tables. One holds the patient demographic information. The second holds the information about the patient's visit, including the clinical department. If the database is stored in flat files, then the clinical department must be added to the first file or the zip code must be added to the second file. If the database is relational, then the two tables may be joined or linked using the patient identifier as a common data element.

In a relational database, the data with a common purpose, concept, or source is arranged into tables. The relationship between the tables is displayed in an entity relationship diagram (ERD). Figure A.1 displays a simple ERD relating a patient information table to a table containing the dates of service for each visit for all patients. This ERD shows that the patient information and visit tables are related by the Patient Identification (Patient ID) variable.

Relational databases are structured in a way that helps ensure data integrity. Notice that in figure A.1, one variable in each table has an icon of a key next to it. These are the primary keys in each of the tables. The primary key uniquely identifies the row in the database. "Patient ID" uniquely identifies a row in the patient information table and "Account Number" uniquely identifies the row in the visits table. Properly defining the primary key field in a table prevents adding of duplicate values of that field in the tables. A foreign key is a variable in one table that is a primary key in another table. In this example, Patient ID is a foreign key in the visits table.

The line extending in figure A.1 from the Patient ID variable in the patient information table to the Patient ID variable in the visits table indicates that these two tables are related

Figure A.1 Entity relationship diagram

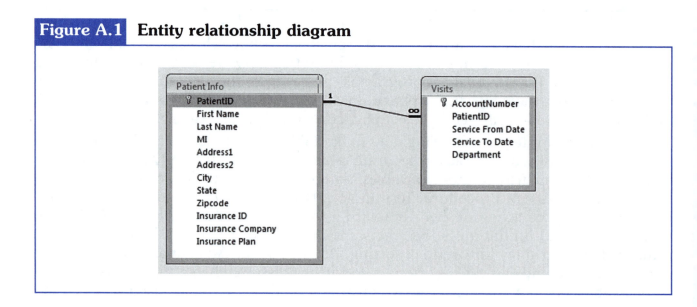

through the Patient ID. Notice that the line has a "1" at the Patient Info table end and the infinity sign (∞) at the Visits table end. These symbols represent the cardinality of the relationship between the two tables. Cardinality for each table refers to the number of elements in each table that are related. Table A.5 presents three types of relationship cardinality in relational databases:

1. One-to-one: Each row in one table relates to one and only one row in the other.
2. One-to-many: Each row in one table may relate to many rows in a second table. Each row in the second table relates to only one row in the first table.
3. Many-to-many: Each row in one table may relate to many rows in a second table; each row in the second table may relate to many rows in the first table.

Table A.5 Cardinality

Cardinality	Table A	Table B	Explanation
One-to-one (1:1)	Patient ID Discharge status code	Discharge status code Definition	Each patient has only one discharge status code; each discharge status code has only one definition
One-to-many (1:N) or (1:∞)	Account number Patient name	Account number Diagnosis code sequence ICD-9-CM diagnosis code	Each account may have many associated diagnosis codes.
Many-to-many (N:N) or (∞:∞)	Account number Bill type Bill date	Account number Bill type Bill date Payment amount	Each account may have multiple bill types and bill dates. Each bill type and bill date may have multiple payments.

Carefully defining the variables in each table and the primary key fields for each table is the first step in ensuring data integrity. Data redundancy or duplication should be avoided in a relational database. The practice of normalization of a database prevents duplication of data elements. There are three forms of normalization:

1. First Normal Form
   a. Eliminate repeating groups in individual tables
   b. Create a separate table for each set of related data
   c. Identify each set of related data with a primary key

2. Second Normal Form
   a. Create separate tables for sets of values that apply to multiple records
   b. Relate these tables with a foreign key

3. Third Normal Form
   a. Eliminate fields that do not depend on the key (Microsoft 2007)

Case Study: Normalizing Data Tables

In this case study, the flat data table included in table A.6 will be converted to a relational database with a normalized form. When data is normalized, the data in one flat file may result in a number of tables.

Table A.6 Normalized data

MRN	Account Number	Date of Service	CDM Item	Revenue Code	Revenue Code Definition	HCPCS Code	Units	Charge
123ABC	1	011011	L01	0300	LABORATORY OR LAB	36415	1	$ 55.75
123ABC	1	011011	L02	0300	LABORATORY OR LAB	84066	1	$ 51.50
123ABC	1	011011	L03	0301	LAB/CHEMISTRY	84153	1	$ 92.25
123ABC	1	011011	C01	0331	CHEMOTHER/INJ	96402	1	$ 168.50
123ABC	1	011011	D01	0636	DRUGS/DETAIL CODE	J9217	1	$ 507.77
987ZYX	2	010411	D02	0250	PHARMACY		6	$ 306.04
987ZYX	2	010411	S01	0270	MED-SUR SUPPLIES		1	$ 11.25
987ZYX	2	010411	S02	0270	MED-SUR SUPPLIES	A6257	1	$ 0.42
987ZYX	2	010411	L04	0305	LAB/HEMATOLOGY	85025	1	$ 107.00
987ZYX	2	010411	C02	0335	CHEMOTHERP-IV	96413	1	$ 495.00
987ZYX	2	010411	E13	0510	CLINIC	99213	1	$ 136.50
987ZYX	2	010411	D03	0636	DRUGS/DETAIL CODE	J2405	8	$ 50.65
987ZYX	2	010411	D04	0636	DRUGS/DETAIL CODE	J9305	100	$ 10,714.56
987ZYX	3	020611	S03	0270	MED-SUR SUPPLIES		1	$ 11.25
987ZYX	3	020611	S02	0270	MED-SUR SUPPLIES	A6257	1	$ 0.42
987ZYX	3	020611	E13	0510	CLINIC	99213	1	$ 136.50

The first normal form requires that the repeating groups are eliminated, separate tables are created for each set of related data, and each resulting table has a primary key. In table A.6, the variables may be segmented into patient information (table A.7) and service information (table A.8).

Table A.7 Patient information

Patient_ID	Account_Number	Service_Date
123ABC	1	1/10/2011
987ZYX	2	01/04/2011
987ZYX	3	02/06/2011

Table A.8 Service information

Services						
Account Number	CDM Item	Revenue Code	Revenue Code Definition	HCPCS Code	Units	Charge
1	L01	0300	LABORATORY OR LAB	36415	1	$ 55.75
1	L02	0300	LABORATORY OR LAB	84066	1	$ 51.50
1	L03	0301	LAB/CHEMISTRY	84153	1	$ 92.25
1	C01	0331	CHEMOTHER/INJ	96402	1	$ 168.50
1	D01	0636	DRUGS/DETAIL CODE	J9217	1	$ 507.77
2	D02	0250	PHARMACY		6	$ 306.04
2	S01	0270	MED-SUR SUPPLIES		1	$ 11.25
2	S02	0270	MED-SUR SUPPLIES	A6257	1	$ 0.42
2	L04	0305	LAB/HEMATOLOGY	85025	1	$ 107.00
2	C02	0335	CHEMOTHERP-IV	96413	1	$ 495.00
2	E13	0510	CLINIC	99213	1	$ 136.50
2	D03	0636	DRUGS/DETAIL CODE	J2405	8	$ 50.65
2	D04	0636	DRUGS/DETAIL CODE	J9305	100	$ 10,714.56
3	S03	0270	MED-SUR SUPPLIES		1	$ 11.25
3	S02	0270	MED-SUR SUPPLIES	A6257	1	$ 0.42
3	E13	0510	CLINIC	99213	1	$ 136.50

The services table may be further broken down into a revenue code definition table, services by account number, and a CDM table. These are displayed in tables A.8a, A.8b, and A.8c.

Table A.8a

Services		
Account Number	CDM Item	Units
1	L01	1
1	L02	1
1	L03	1
1	C01	1
1	D01	1
2	D02	6
2	S01	1
2	S02	1
2	L04	1
2	C02	1
2	E13	1
2	D03	8
2	D04	100
3	S03	1
3	S02	1
3	E13	1

Table A.8b

Charge Description Master			
CDM Item	Revenue Code	HCPCS Code	Unit Charge
C01	0331	96402	168.50
C02	0335	96413	495.00
D01	0636	J9217	507.77
D02	0250		51.01
D03	0636	J2405	6.33
D04	0636	J9305	107.15
E13	0510	99213	136.50
L01	0300	36415	55.75
L02	0300	84066	51.50
L03	0301	84153	92.25
L04	0305	85025	107.00
S01	0270		11.25
S02	0270	A6257	0.42
S03	0270		11.25

Table A.8c

Revenue Codes	
Revenue Code	Revenue Code Definition
0250	PHARMACY
0270	MED-SUR SUPPLIES
0300	LABORATORY OR LAB
0301	LAB/ CHEMISTRY
0305	LAB/ HEMATOLOGY
0331	CHEMOTHER/ INJ
0335	CHEMOTHERP-IV
0510	CLINIC
0363	DRUGS/DETAIL CODE

The final step in first order normalization is to identify the primary key fields in each table. The primary key for the visits table is account number. The primary key in table A.8a is a combination of the account number and the CDM item. The primary key in table A.8b is the CDM item and finally, the primary key in the table A.8c is the revenue code.

While eliminating repeating rows, the tables now actually also conform to the second normalized form. Recall that the second normalized form requires that separate tables are created for sets of values that apply to multiple records and that the tables are related with a foreign key.

The ERD displayed in figure A.2 shows the relationships between the normalized tables. Notice that the field names were converted to single words by inserting an underscore between the words in the original variable names. It is best practice to use single word variable or field names and table names to simplify the syntax for writing queries and reports.

The final step in normalization is to check the third normalized form. To conform to the third normalized form, all fields that do not depend on a key (primary or foreign) must be eliminated. The tables in figure A.2 do not include any fields that do not depend on the key fields and therefore the tables are completely normalized.

Figure A.2 **Relationships between normalized tables**

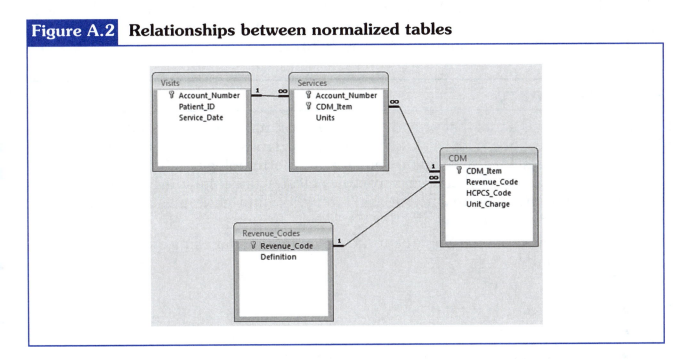

Object-Oriented Databases

Object-oriented databases are designed to handle data types beyond text and numbers. Flat file and relational databases were developed to store data that fits into rows and columns. Object-oriented databases may be used to store images or videos. In healthcare, object-oriented databases may be used to store images from a magnetic resonance imaging (MRI), x-ray, or even an audio file capturing the heartbeat heard during a prenatal ultrasound. The building blocks of an object-oriented database are the objects as opposed to tables in a relational database system.

An object-oriented database stores two types of information about the object. The first element is the data itself (audio clip, image, video file, and such). The second element stored describes how to use the data and is called the method. Object-oriented databases are currently not used widely in practice, but the expansion of the EHR will require the storage of many objects beyond the simple rows and columns of numbers and text that may be stored in relational databases.

Database Management Software

To access and manipulate a database, it must reside in a software tool. The choice of database software depends on the type of database, the size of the database, and the complexity of the relationships between the database elements. Relational databases are found most often in practice. The most common relational database software applications include Microsoft Access, Oracle, and Microsoft Structured Query Language (SQL) Server.

Microsoft Access is typically run on a workstation and is appropriate for smaller department-specific applications. It is also useful for prototyping larger enterprise-wide database systems. Once the number of users expands and Access can no longer efficiently accommodate the database, the database may require a more sophisticated software application. Microsoft offers a wizard that allows users to convert an Access database to a SQL Server database (Microsoft 2011).

Data Dictionary

A data dictionary is a tool that provides metadata, or information about data. Metadata is defined as data about data. A key focus of a data dictionary is to support and adopt more consistent use of data elements and terminology to improve the use of data in reporting. A data dictionary promotes clearer understanding; helps users find information; promotes more efficient use or reuse of information; and promotes better data management (Bronnert et al. 2011, 5).

A data dictionary should document the following attributes of the fields in a data table at a minimum:

- Field name
- Table name
- Description of the field
- Data type (numeric, text, or field length)
- Data frequency (required field or not)
- Is the field a primary or foreign key?
- Valid values
- Data source
- Field creation date
- Field termination date
- Update frequency

The data dictionary in table A.9 documents the contents of the CDM table found in the normalization example. The details included in this table allow a user with little or no knowledge of the contents of the table to understand the fields present and their various roles.

Table A.9 Data dictionary

Field Name	Table	Description	Data Type	Field Length	Data Frequency	Key?	Valid Values	Data Source	Field Creation Date	Field Termination Date	Update Frequency
CDM Item	CDM	CDM Item code	Text	20	Required	Primary	Alpha-numeric	Fianace	1/1/1900		N/A
Revenue Code	CDM	UB-04 revenue code	Text	4	Required	Foreign	Valid revenue code	HIM	1/1/1900		Annual
HCPCS Code	CDM	CPT/HCPCS level II	Text	5		Foreign	Valid HCPCS	HIM	1/1/1900		Annual
Unit Charge	CDM	Charge per unit	Currency	10	Required		>=$0.00	Finance	1/1/1900		Annaul

Structured Query Language (SQL)

Structured Query Language (SQL) is the programming language that is used to manipulate data in a relational database. SQL is sometimes pronounced sequel or S. Q. L. SQL fulfills many roles in a DBMS:

- SQL is an interactive query language. Users type SQL commands into an interactive SQL program to retrieve data and display it on the screen, providing a convenient, easy-to-use tool for ad hoc database queries.

- SQL is a database programming language. Programmers embed SQL commands into their application programs to access the data in a database. Both user written programs and database utility programs (such as report writers and data entry tools) use this technique for database access.

- SQL is a database administration language. The database administrator responsible for managing a minicomputer or mainframe database uses SQL to define the database structure and control access to the stored data.

- SQL is a client or server language. Personal computer programs use SQL to communicate over a network with database servers that store shared data. This client or server architecture has become very popular for enterprise-class applications.

- SQL is an internet data access language. Internet web servers that interact with corporate data and internet applications servers all use SQL as a standard language for accessing corporate databases.

- SQL is a distributed database language. Distributed DBMSs use SQL to help distribute data across many connected computer systems. The DBMS software on each system uses SQL to communicate with the other systems, sending requests for data access.

- SQL is a database gateway language. In a computer network with a mix of different DBMS products, SQL is often used in a gateway that allows one brand of DBMS to communicate with another brand (Groff et al. 2010, 6).

The role of SQL as an interactive query language is described in more detail in the following section. Health information management (HIM) professionals should be aware that SQL is far more than just a tool used to extract data from a relational database.

SQL commands used to retrieve data follow a basic structure that allows non-programmers to understand and write queries. For example, a SQL command to collect all of the visits for a particular patient in the visits table found in table A.7 is:

SELECT * FROM visits WHERE patient_id = '987ZYX'

The results of the query are the two records displayed in table A.10.

Table A.10 **Select query**

Account_Number	Patient_ID	Service_Date
2	987ZYX	1/4/2011
3	987ZYX	2/6/2011

This is called a select query. The purpose of a select query is to pull records that meet a certain criteria from a particular table or combination of tables. The letters in the words SELECT, FROM, and WHERE are capitalized in the query because they represent key words or instructions in the SQL command.

In this case, the two visit records for patient 987ZYX were selected from the three records found in the visits table (see Table A.7 for the three patient records). The query may be modified to present the records in a particular order. For instance, the records in the previous example may be sorted by descending service date by revising the query to include an ORDER BY statement:

> SELECT Visits.Account_Number, Visits.Patient_ID, Visits.Service_Date
>
> FROM Visits
>
> WHERE Visits.Patient_ID)="987ZYX"
>
> ORDER BY Visits.Service_Date DESC;

The ORDER BY clause states that the results of the query should be sorted by descending service date. The results of this query are presented in table A.11.

Table A.11 Select query example results

Account_Number	Patient_ID	Service_Date
3	987ZYX	2/6/2011
2	987ZYX	1/4/2011

A select query may be used to combine data from two or more tables by defining a join. For example, a SQL query to select all of the patients that received the medical supply with the CDM item code equal to S02 would require the services table be joined to the visits table. The relationship between these tables is found in the ERD displayed in figure A.2. The tables must be combined or joined based on the account_number field. When more than one table is included in a query, the fields are references by both the table and field name concatenated together and delimited by a period. For example, when referring to the field account_number in the visits table, the user would reference the field as visits.account_number. The following select query will find the patients who received CDM item S02:

> SELECT Visits.Account_Number, Visits.Patient_ID, Visits.Service_Date, Services.CDM_Item, Services.Units
>
> FROM Visits INNER JOIN Services ON Visits.Account_Number = Services.Account_Number
>
> WHERE Services.CDM_Item="S02"

In this query, the SELECT statement includes the fields that are desired; the FROM statement includes the two tables (Visits and Services) as well as how those two tables should be related (Account_Number). Finally, the WHERE statement indicates that only rows where the CDM_Item is equal to S02 in the Services table. The results of this query are presented in table A.12.

Table A.12 Join query example results

Account_Number	Patient_ID	Service_Date	CDM_Item	Units
2	987ZYX	1/4/2011	S02	1
3	987ZYX	2/6/2011	S02	1

A SQL command may also be used to summarize data. In the above example, a count of the number of visits for each patient may be generated with the following query:

```
SELECT Visits.Patient_ID, Count(Visits.Service_Date) AS CountOfService_Date
FROM Visits
GROUP BY Visits.Patient_ID;
```

This query includes the familiar SELECT and FROM keywords, but notice that there is now also a GROUP BY statement. When a query is used to summarize data, the summary statistic and the field that designates the group to be summarized must be designated. In the example, the SELECT statement includes a command that creates a count of the number of service dates (Count(Visits.Service_Date)) and stores that result in a new field called CountOfService_Date. The GROUP BY portion of the query states that the counts should be presented by Patient_ID. The result of this query is presented in table A.13.

Table A.13 Count of service dates

Patient_ID	CountOfService_Date
123ABC	1
987ZYX	2

There are a number of excellent online resources that can be helpful in learning more about SQL commands. A search using the terms SQL or SQL basics will yield many tutorials and references.

Data Modeling

A data model is a representation of the data to be stored in a database and the relationships between the tables and data fields. Prior to the design of the database, the business process to be supported by the database must be modeled. This may be accomplished through the use of process and data flow diagrams. The components of a database discussed previously in this chapter is designed and assembled in a way that supports the business process requirements. Data modeling may be carried out using either an object-oriented or entity relationship approach. The entity relationship approach will be outlined here.

There are two important outputs to the data modeling process. First, the ERD is a graphical representation of the tables in the database and their relationships. The second output is the data dictionary. Both of these documents were discussed earlier in this chapter. The data model serves as the basis for the database structure and design as documented by the ERD and data dictionary.

The process of data modeling includes three steps: the conceptual model, the logical model, and the physical data model. The conceptual model includes a mapping of the business requirements for the database using non technical terms that end users can understand. A database that does not meet the need of the end users is of no value, so they must be involved in the design process at the earliest stage. The conceptual data model is independent of the type of database that will ultimately be used to store the data. The conceptual data model may be mapped using a context-level data flow diagram which maps out the database's boundary and scope. Figure A.3 shows a context-level data flow diagram for the claims database example used earlier in this chapter. Notice that the diagram does not include any field or table information. It simply displays the general categories of data and their roles in the business process. The details regarding the actual database structure are fleshed out in the logical modeling step.

The logical model is the next step in database modeling. During this phase the tables start to take shape. The fields are not defined, but the basic contents of the tables and how they relate are defined. In our claims data example, the tables are as follows:

- Patient information
- Visit for each patient
- Services provided to patient
- Charge for services

The relationships between the tables may be mapped out in a Diagram 0 data flow diagram. A Diagram 0 data flow diagram expands on the context diagram and adds details regarding the tables and their relationships. Figure A.4 displays a Diagram 0 for the claims database example.

The final step in the database modeling process is to determine the physical model. This includes mapping out the tables, keys, and relationships using an ERD, as well as determining the DBMS and hardware to house the database. The ERD for this example

---

Figure A.3   **Context-level data flow diagram**

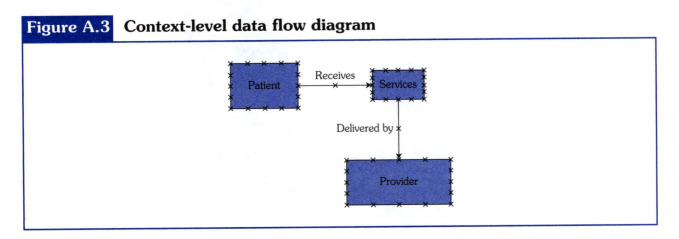

is displayed in figure A.2. At this point in the modeling process, a database type may be selected. Since this database requires multiple tables that may need to be linked together for reporting purposes, a relational database is the best choice for this business process. There are a number of DBMSs that support relational database structures including the following:

- Microsoft Access
- Microsoft SQL Server
- Informix
- Oracle
- MySQL

The choice of specific DBMS software should be based on the size and scope of the database as well as the budget for the project. Microsoft Access is an excellent choice for small departmental databases, but is not suited for enterprise-wide databases with many users because the administration of user access at various levels is not possible. Oracle is an extremely robust DBMS and can accommodate very complex models with many users. Oracle licenses tend to be significantly more expensive than Microsoft Access. For this reason, departmental-level databases are often maintained in Access. There are some open-source DBMS that are free to the public, but may not have the support network that some of the commercial products have.

The physical model also includes a specification of the computer hardware that will be used to house the database. The amount of storage or disk space required for the database should be determined prior to selecting any hardware platform. Estimating the space required for the database currently and for the foreseeable future will help

Figure A.4   **Diagram 0**

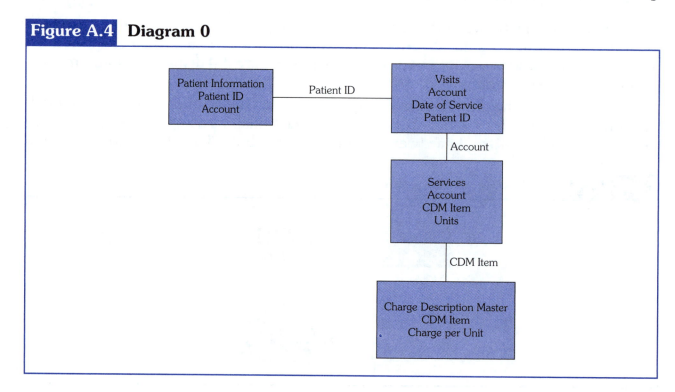

determine the appropriate hardware and software to select for implementation of the database.

Clinical Data Warehouses

Clinical databases are found throughout healthcare operations. The example in this chapter was a very simple database designed to hold information about the services provided to a patient. Clinical databases may be found in various departments throughout a healthcare facility, including:

- Patient accounting
- Clinical departments
- Pharmacy
- Clinical trials
- Marketing
- Quality measurement

Combining these data sources into a clinical data warehouse is an effective method of making the data accessible to a wider audience of users. A clinical data warehouse must be designed in a way that maintains sufficient detail so that the data is useful for research and analytic purposes and related in a way that supports real-time access to the data by users. Data warehouses are snapshots of a variety of databases found throughout a company that are combined for the purpose of reporting and analysis. The data warehouse does not include the live or transaction data that are used for business operations, but instead are populated by periodic downloads from the live database. The frequency of the refreshing the clinical data warehouse depends on the volatility of the underlying data (how often it changes) and the need for timely reporting.

The Stanford School of Medicine has an extensive clinical data warehouse called STRIDE (Stanford Translational Research Integrated Database Environment) that stores data that supports clinical and translational research (Stanford Center for Clinical Informatics 2012). STRIDE includes data from both hospitals affiliated with Stanford. The hospitals use different billing systems and yet the warehouse is designed to combine the datasets across the facilities. As of January 2013, the STRIDE warehouse included the following datasets:

- 1.85 million pediatric and adult patients with clinical and demographic data (1994–present)
- 21.5 million Clinical Encounters (1994–present)
- 40 million ICD-9-coded inpatient and outpatient diagnoses (1994–present)
- 25 million ICD-9 and CPT-coded inpatient and outpatient clinical procedures (1994–present)
- 3.1 million radiology reports (2005–present)
- 1.3 million surgical pathology reports (1995–present)
- 21 million transcribed clinical documents (2005–present)

- 145 million laboratory test numeric results (2000–present)
- 14 million inpatient pharmacy orders (2006–present)
- 99,000 dates of death drawn from hospital and Social Security Administration records

Clinical data warehouses like Stanford's STRIDE are becoming widespread as the technology to support the storage and access of huge volumes of data.

Decision support databases are a common example of a clinical data warehouse. These databases are found in many healthcare entities and may include claims data, financial data, and quality data combined in one database to support both internal and external reporting. One of the unique challenges in combining clinical data is that any release of that data may be subject to HIPAA regulations if it includes any of the protected health information fields such as dates or Social Security numbers. Any efforts to combine data into a clinical data warehouse should include the involvement of a compliance officer or other professional with knowledge of the rules and regulations surrounding deidentification of data and the release of identifiable data.

Much of the time and effort invested in compiling a clinical data warehouse is used to clean and combine the data. Although clinical data is singularly focused on healthcare and patient information, the coding systems may or may not be consistent. For instance, pharmacy databases may include National Drug Code (NDC) or may only include an inventory or CDM code that only has meaning inside a particular facility or system of facilities. The mapping between code sets and standardization of coding systems is an age-old issue in healthcare data. Many thought that the HIPAA regulations specifying only one coding system for each purpose would solve this problem. The concept of common ontology, or system of categories, as a method of combining data that may be categorized by clinical classification systems such as ICD and CPT codes as well as those categorized by clinical nomenclatures such as Systematized Nomenclature Of Medicine Clinical Terms (SNOMED). According to Smith and Ceusters, an effective ontology is "a theory of those higher-level categories which structure the biomedical domain, the representation of which needs to be both unified and coherent if it is to serve as the basis for terminologies and coding systems that have the requisite degree and type of interoperability" (2007). A properly designed ontology may allow the automated combining of data from many sources. Such a system would speed the design and delivery of new clinical data warehouses.

✎ Summary

Understanding the basic structure and guidelines for database design is a critical skill for health information and informatics professionals. Healthcare has a wealth of data that must be organized in a way that allows accurate and efficient processing and reporting. The type of database selected for a business process should be based on the level of complexity of the relationships between the data.

Many database concepts are applicable across the spectrum of database types. The design of the database through the stages of data modeling is as necessary when designing a flat file to hold data with a relatively simple structure as it is when designing an object-oriented database that holds multimedia files as well as numeric and text format data. Data dictionaries are also useful for all database types. Without documentation to inform the user of the format, type, and definitions of data elements the data may not be used for reporting. The basic SQL commands covered in this chapter are transferable across a variety of DBMSs for relational databases. There are slight syntax differences between the various database software products, but the basic structure and key words are transferable across products.

References

Bronnert, J., J. Clark, L. Hyde, J. Solberg, S. White, and M. Wolin. 2011. *Health Data Analysis Toolkit*. Chicago: AHIMA.

Codd, E.F. 1970. A relational model of data for large shared data banks. Edited by P. Baxendate *Communications of the ACM*, 13(6):377–387.

Groff, J., P. Weinberg, and A. Oppel. 2010. *SQL: The Complete Reference*, 3rd ed. New York: McGraw-Hill/Osborne.

Microsoft. 2007. Description of the Database Normalization Basics. http://support.microsoft.com/kb/283878

Microsoft. 2011. How to Convert an Access Database to SQL Server. http://support.microsoft.com/kb/237980

Smith, B and W. Ceusters. 2007. Ontology as the Core Discipline of Biomedical Informatics: Legacies of the Past and Recommendations for the Future Direction of Research. Chapter 7 in *Computing, Philosophy, and Cognitive Science: The Nexus and the Liminal*. Edited by Dodig-Crnkovic, G. and S. Stuart. Cambridge: Cambridge Scholars Press.

Stanford Center for Clinical Informatics. 2012. Clinical Data Warehouse Projects - SCCI Stanford Medicine. https://clinicalinformatics.stanford.edu/projects/cdw.html

Resources

Brazhnik, O., and J. Jones. 2007. Anatomy of data integration. *Journal of Biomedical Informatics* 40(3): 252–269.

Gibas C. and P. Jambeck 2001. *Developing Bioinformatics Computer Skills*. Sebastopol: O'Reilly Media, Inc.

Shelly, R. 2010. *Systems Analysis and Design*. Boston: Cengage Course Technology.

Appendix B: Excel Data Analysis Reference

Native Excel Statistical Functions

Excel 2010 includes a number of functions that are useful for performing statistical analysis.

A full listing of the native Excel functions for statistical analysis may be found at this website:

http://office.microsoft.com/en-us/excel-help/statistical-functions-HP005203066.aspx?CTT=3

This link includes a full listing of all of the statistical functions, the types of arguments they require, and examples of how to implement the functions.

About the Excel Data Analysis ToolPak

The Data Analysis ToolPak (DAT) is an Excel Add-in that extends the statistical analysis functionality of Excel. The DAT uses the native Excel functions for the calculations, but packages many of them together to allow a user to perform basic descriptive and inferential statistics in one step. The DAT is available in the Windows versions of Excel from 2007 on. Unfortunately, Microsoft opted to remove the DAT from the Mac version of Excel in 2008. Microsoft recommends a product called StatPlus: mac LE as a replacement. StatPlus: mac LE may be downloaded for free from this link: http://www.analystsoft.com/en/products/statplusmacle/. This reference guide will cover the Windows version of the DAT, but many of the concepts found here are transferable to the Mac product. The native statistical functions listed in the previous section are available in both the Windows and Mac versions of Excel.

Installing the Data Analysis ToolPak

The DAT is included with all Excel licenses except the starter versions. The DAT is not available to the user until it is activated. To check to see if the DAT is activated, open Excel and click "Data" on the main menu bar (top of the screen). If "Data Analysis" is present in the ribbon menu as depicted in figure B.1, then the DAT is active.

Figure B.1 Ribbon menu

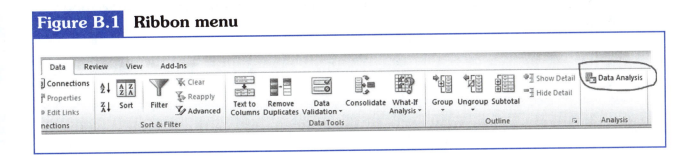

If the DAT is not active then perform the following steps:

Step 1: Click "File" on the main menu

Step 2: Click "Options"

Step 3: Click "Add-ins"

Step 4: Select "Excel Add-ins" from the drop down menu to the right of the word Manage at the bottom of the screen

Step 5: Click "Go" (see figure B.2)

Figure B.2 **Step 4 and step 5**

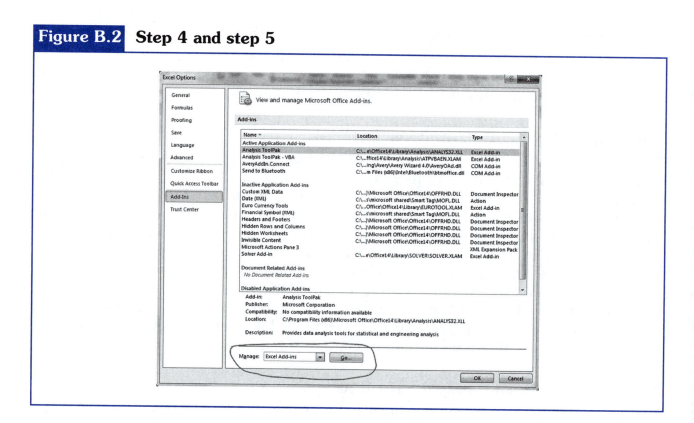

Step 6: Click the check box for Analysis ToolPak and Analysis ToolPak - VBA (see figure B.3).

Step 7: Click "OK"

Step 8: Check to see if the Data Analysis option is present on the data ribbon as shown in figure A.1.

Figure B.3 | **Step 6**

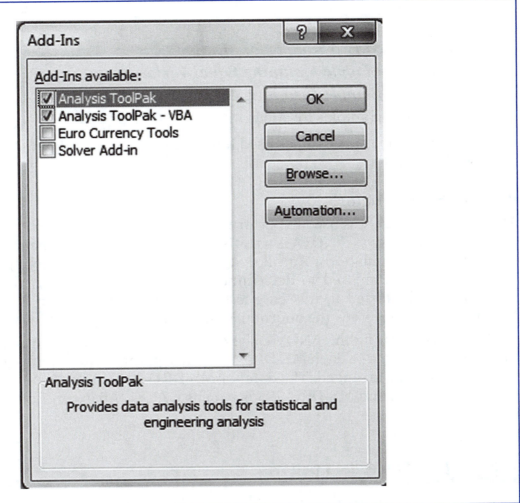

Using the Data Analysis ToolPak

The DAT includes the following 19 choices:

- ***Anova: Single Factor***
- Anova: Two-Factor with Replication
- Anova: Two-Factor without Replication
- ***Correlation***
- Covariance
- ***Descriptive Statistics***
- Exponential Smoothing
- ***F-Test Two Sample for Variance***
- Fourier Analysis
- ***Histogram***
- Moving Average
- ***Random Number Generation***

- Rank and Percentile
- *Regression*
- Sampling
- t-*Test: Paired Two Sample for Means*
- t-*Test: Two-Sample Assuming Equal Variances*
- t-*Test: Two-Sample Assuming Unequal Variances*
- Z-Test: Two-Samples for Mean

This guide reviews the choices used in this text (denoted in ***bold italics***) in the order presented in Excel.

ANOVA: Single Factor

ANOVA: Single Factor is used to perform a one-way analysis of variance as presented in chapter 5. The one-way ANOVA is a statistical inference method that is used to compare more than two populations. Recall that in example 5.11, the charge per case for three MS-DRGs were compared to determine if they were statistically different. The null hypothesis to be tested in this case is that the population mean charge for all three MS-DRGs is equal versus the alternative that at least one pair of means is not equal.

Prior to performing the ANOVA, the data must be arranged so that the charges for the patients assigned to each MS-DRG are in a separate column. Figure B.4 shows how the data should be arranged. The data for MS-DRG 291 is in cells A2:A81, MS-DRG 292 is in cells B2:B81, and MS-DRG 293 is in cells C2:C81. An excerpt of this data is shown in Figure B.4.

Figure B.4 **ANOVA data pattern**

	A	B	C
1	MS-DRG 291	MS-DRG 292	MS-DRG 293
2	21426	164904	35255
3	70379	79101	15039
4	102111	62293	13801
5	71078	39438	43325
6	23928	36438	25213
7	20134	27710	6085
8	30819	23253	46655
9	66705	21687	38028
10	43929	13254	26963
11	36968	8845	28532

To create the ANOVA table, click "Data" on the main menu and then click "Data Analysis" on the data ribbon. The window in figure A.5 should appear. Select "ANOVA: Single Factor" and then click "OK."

Figure B.6 shows the ANOVA: Single Factor window populated for the example data.

| **Figure B.5** | **Data analysis window** |

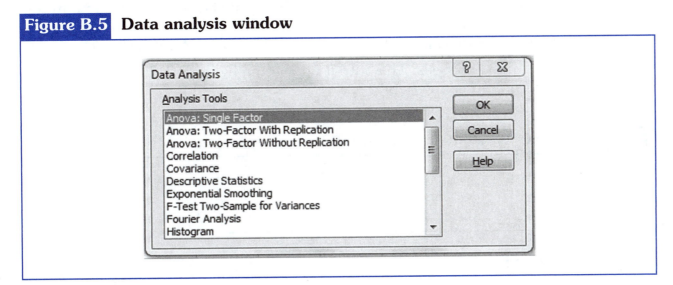

| **Figure B.6** | **ANOVA: single factor window** |

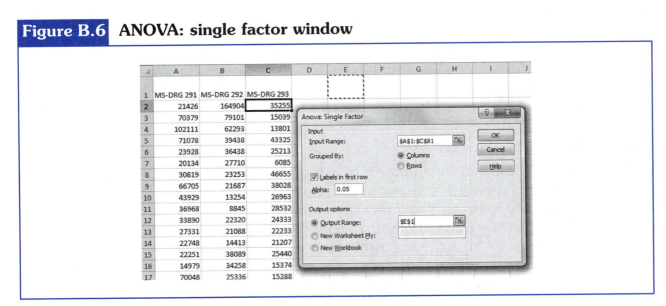

The data elements required are as follows:

1. Input range: The data appears in A1:C81. Notice that the data input range starts in row 1 so that the labels for the groups can be included in the output. You may highlight the range of the worksheet you wish to include, or type it in using a $ sign before column and row labels and separating upper left and lower right cell names with a colon, for example, $A$1:$C$81.

2. Grouped by: The groups are in each column. The data could be transposed so that the groups are represented by rows. If that is the case, then the row radio button should be selected.

3. Labels in first row: Check this box if the data in the input range includes the data labels in the first row. This tells Excel to use the first row as titles and not actual data values.

4. Alpha: This is the alpha level for the hypothesis test to be performed.

5. Output options: The location options for the output should be presented. In this example, the output will be placed starting in cell E1 of the current worksheet. The output may also be placed in a new worksheet or a new workbook.

Click "OK" to run the analysis. The output appears in figure B.7. The interpretation of this output was presented in chapter 5.

Figure B.7 ANOVA: single factor output

Anova: Single Factor

SUMMARY

Groups	Count	Sum	Average	Variance
MS-DRG 291	80	3,550,238	44,378	733,847,198
MS-DRG 292	80	2,609,870	32,623	572,536,931
MS-DRG 293	80	1,890,221	23,628	123,870,483

ANOVA

Source of Variation	SS	df	MS	F	P-value	F crit
Between Groups	17,324,346,245	2	8,662,173,123	18.169	0.000	3.034
Within Groups	112,990,114,407	237	476,751,538			
Total	130,314,460,653	239				

Correlation

Correlation was presented in chapter 6 as a method of measuring the strength of the linear relationship between two variables. The Excel correlation function presents the Pearson's r correlation only and therefore should only be used when measuring the correlation between two interval or ratio variables. The data should be arranged so that the columns represent the variables and the rows represent the subjects. The data from example 6.1 in the text will be used to demonstrate the correlation function in the DAT.

Select "Data" from the main menu and then click "Data Analysis" on the data ribbon. Figure A.8 shows the data analysis menu with "Correlation" selected. Click "OK" after selecting "Correlation."

Figure B.9 shows the correlation window populated for the example data. The data elements required are as follows:

1. Input range: The data appears in B1:C8. Notice that the data input range starts in row 1 so that the labels for the groups can be included in the output. The column representing the subject identifier is not included in the input range.

Figure B.8   Data analysis window

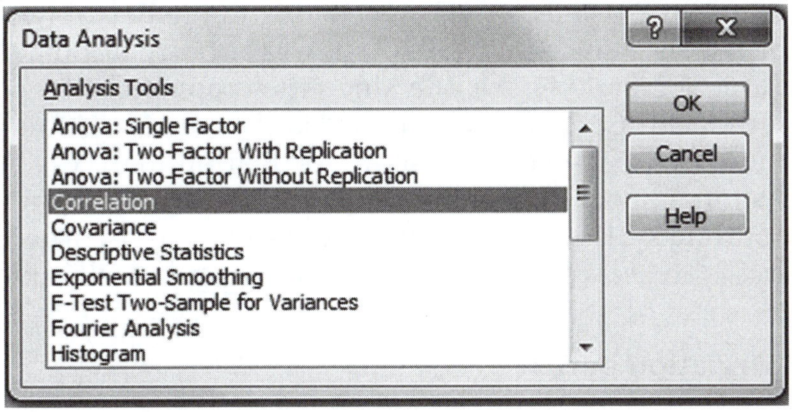

Figure B.9   Correlation window

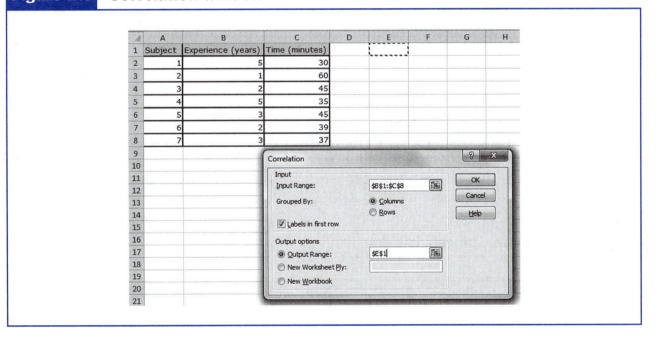

2. Grouped by: The variables are in each column. The data could be transposed so that the variables are represented by rows. If that is the case, then the row radio button should be selected.

3. Labels in first row: Check this box if the data in the input range includes the data labels in the first row. This tells Excel to use the first row as titles and not actual data values.

4. Output options: The location for the output should be presented. In this example, the output will be placed starting in cell E1 of the current worksheet. The output may also be placed in a new worksheet or a new workbook.

Click "OK" to run the analysis. The output appears in figure B.10. The interpretation of this output was presented in chapter 6.

The output that appears in cells E1:G3 is a correlation matrix. The first row and first column are variable labels. Notice that cell F3 shows the correlation between experience and coding time. Cells F2 and G3 are one since they represent the correlation of one of the variables with itself. Cell G2 is blank, but is the same value as F3. The order of the variables does not matter in correlation. A correlation matrix is always symmetric across the main diagonal of one. The main diagonal starts in the upper left hand corner of a matrix and continues diagonally to the lower right hand corner. In a correlation matrix, this represents the correlation of each variable with itself and is always one.

Figure B.10 **Correlation output**

	E	F	G
1		Experience (years)	Time (minutes)
2	Experience (years)	1	
3	Time (minutes)	-0.830047203	1

Descriptive Statistics

Descriptive statistics for continuous variables was presented in chapter 5. The data for example 5.1 in the text is used to demonstrate the functionality of the descriptive statistics function in the DAT. Select "Data" from the main menu and then click "Data Analysis" on the data ribbon. Figure A.11 shows the Data Analysis menu with "Descriptive Statistics" selected. Click "OK" after selecting "Descriptive Statistics."

Figure B.11 **Data analysis window**

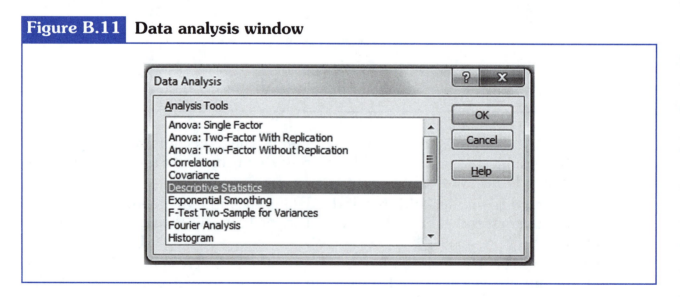

Figure B.12 Descriptive statistics window

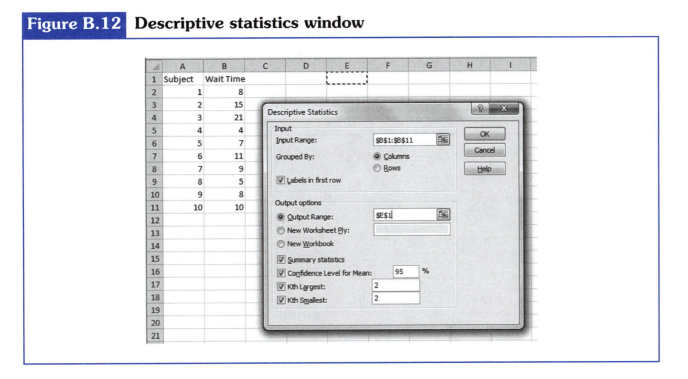

Figure B.12 shows the descriptive statistics window populated for the example data. The data elements required are as follows:

1. **Input range:** The data appears in B1:B11. Notice that the data input range starts in row 1 so that the labels for the groups can be included in the output. The column representing the subject identifier is not included in the input range.

2. **Grouped by:** The variables are in each column. The data could be transposed so that the variables are represented by rows. If that is the case, then the row radio button should be selected.

3. **Labels in first row:** Check this box if the data in the input range includes the data labels in the first row. This tells Excel to use the first row as titles and not actual data values.

4. **Output options:** The location for the output should be presented. In this example, the output will be placed starting in cell E1 of the current worksheet. The output may also be placed in a new worksheet or a new workbook.

5. **Summary statistics:** Check this box so that the output includes summary statistics.

6. **Confidence level for mean:** Check this box and enter a value for the confidence level. The output will then include the width of a confidence interval at the designated level.

7. **Kth largest:** Check this box to include the largest values in the output. Input the number of largest values to include in the output. This example used the value two, so the value next to the maximum value will appear in the output.

8. **Kth smallest:** Check this box to include the smallest values in the output. Input the number of smallest values to include in the output. This example used the value two, so the value next to the minimum value will appear in the output.

Note that the Kth largest and smallest values are useful when trying to determine if there are any gross outliers or extreme values in the data set. Click "OK" to run the analysis. The output appears in figure B.10. The interpretation of this output was presented in chapter 6.

Figure B.13 | **Descriptive statistics output**

	A	B	C	D	E	F
1	Subject	Wait Time			Wait Time	
2	1	8				
3	2	15			Mean	9.8
4	3	21			Standard Error	1.583246
5	4	4			Median	8.5
6	5	7			Mode	8
7	6	11			Standard Deviation	5.006662
8	7	9			Sample Variance	25.06667
9	8	5			Kurtosis	1.987299
10	9	8			Skewness	1.336251
11	10	10			Range	17
12					Minimum	4
13					Maximum	21
14					Sum	98
15					Count	10
16					Largest(2)	15
17					Smallest(2)	5
18					Confidence Level(95.0%)	3.58155
19						

Click "OK" to run the analysis. The output appears in figure B.13. The interpretation of most of the statistics presented was reviewed in chapter 5. The definitions of kurtosis and skewness were not included in chapter 6. Skewness measures how symmetric the values of a variable are with respect to the mean. Skewness close to zero means that the variable is symmetric around the mean. Kurtosis is a measure of how closely grouped the data values are around the mean. These two statistics are used to assess how close the distribution of a variable is to the normal distribution. The normal distribution has a skewness of 0 and a kurtosis of three. In this case, the wait times are not normally distributed.

The output labeled "Confidence Level" (95.0 percent) is the half-width of a 95 percent confidence interval for the population mean wait times. This can be combined with the sample mean to formulate the confidence interval: 9.8 ± 3.6 or (6.2 minutes, 13.4 minutes)

F-Test Two-Sample for Variances

The F-test two-sample for variances performs an hypothesis test for the equality of two variances. Two-sample t-tests were presented in chapter 5 as a method for comparing two population means. There are two formulations of the two-sample t-test. One formula is appropriate when the two population variances are assumed to be equal and a second formula is appropriate if that assumption is not made. Figure 5.3 shows the Statistical Product and Service Solutions (SPSS) output for the two-sample t-test that includes the test for equality of variances. SPSS uses Levene's test for the equality of two variances. The Excel DAT uses the F-test to test the hypothesis, but it must be run separately from the two-sample t-test. The data for example 5.9 is used to demonstrate the F-test two-sample for variances. In this example, the average charge for patients admitted through the emergency department is compared to the average charge for patients not admitted through the emergency department. The null hypothesis for the F-test is that the two population variances are equal. The alternative hypothesis is that they are unequal.

Select "Data" from the main menu and then click "Data Analysis" on the data ribbon. Figure B.14 shows the Data Analysis menu with F-test two-sample for variances selected. Click "OK" after selecting "F-Test Two-Sample for Variances."

Figure B.14 **Data analysis window**

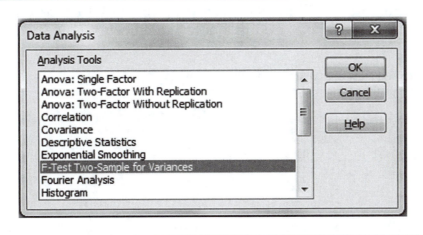

Figure B.15 **F-test two-sample for variance window**

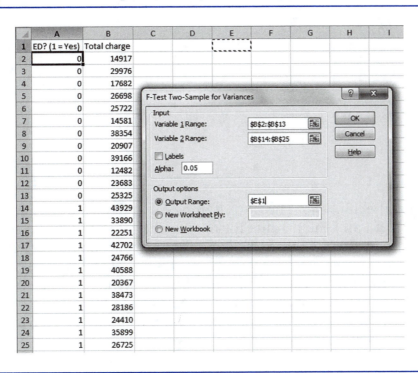

Figure B.15 shows the F-test two-sample for variances window populated for the example data. The data elements required are as follows:

1. Variable one range: The data appears in B2:B13.

2. Variable two range: The data appears in B14:B25.

3. Labels in first row: Check this box if the data in the input range includes the data labels in the first row. This tells Excel to use the first row as titles and not actual data values. Since the data is stacked in the same column, the label is not included in the range and this check box is unchecked.

4. Alpha: This is the alpha level for the test of the null hypothesis that the two population variances are equal.

5. Output options: The location options for the output should be presented. In this example, the output will be placed starting in cell E1 of the current worksheet. The output may also be placed in a new worksheet or a new workbook.

Figure B.16 **F-test two-sample variance output**

	A	B	C	D	E	F	G
1	ED? (1 = Yes)	Total charge			F-Test Two-Sample for Variances		
2	0	14917					
3	0	29976				Variable 1	Variable 2
4	0	17682			Mean	24124.41667	31848.83333
5	0	26698			Variance	76094440.27	70333469.97
6	0	25722			Observations	12	12
7	0	14581			df	11	11
8	0	38354			F	1.081909371	
9	0	20907			P(F<=f) one-tail	0.449229269	
10	0	39166			F Critical one-tail	2.81793047	
11	0	12482					
12	0	23683					
13	0	25325					
14	1	43929					
15	1	33890					
16	1	22251					
17	1	42702					
18	1	24766					
19	1	40588					
20	1	20367					
21	1	38473					
22	1	28186					
23	1	24410					
24	1	35899					
25	1	26725					

Click "OK" to run the analysis. The output appears in figure B.16. The output presents the F test value (1.08) and the p-value for testing the hypothesis that the two variances are equal. In this case, the p-value is 0.45 which is larger than our pre specified alpha of 0.05. Therefore, we do not reject the null hypothesis that the two population variances are equal. Notice that the F-test statistic used by Excel is different from Levene's test for the same null hypothesis. In this case, both tests yield the same conclusion. Levene's test performs better when the data is non normal. Excel does not have the functionality to perform Levene's test built into the DAT.

Histogram

A histogram is an excellent tool to use in describing the distribution of the values of a variable. A histogram was used in chapter 6 to determine if the standardized residuals from a simple linear regression were approximately normally distributed. The histogram function in the DAT will be demonstrated using the standardized residuals from example 6.5 from the text.

Select "Data" from the main menu and then click "Data Analysis" on the data ribbon. Figure B.17 shows the data analysis menu with "Histogram" selected. Click "OK" after selecting "Histogram."

Figure B.17 **Data analysis window**

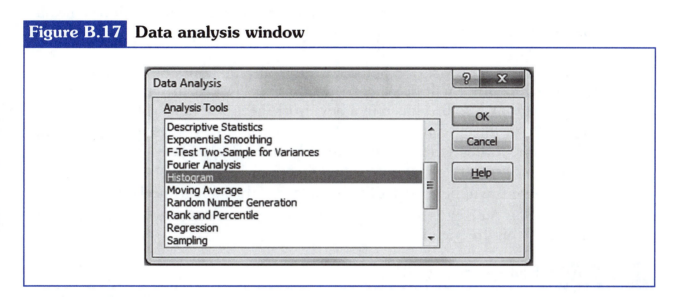

Figure B.18 **Histogram window**

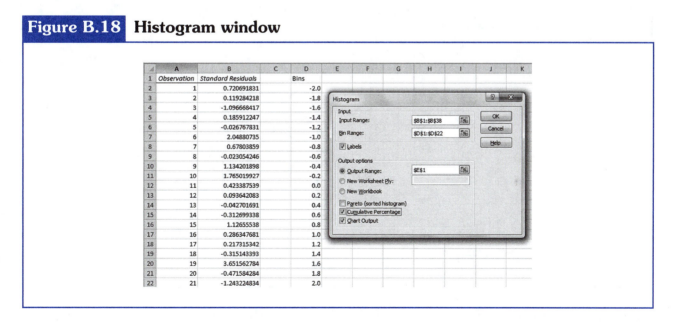

Figure B.18 shows the histogram window populated for the example data. The data elements required are as follows:

1. **Input range:** The data appears in B1:B38. Notice that the data input range starts in row 1 so that the labels for the groups can be included in the output. The column representing the subject identifier is not included in the input range.

2. **Bin range:** A histogram reports the frequency of observations within ranges. The bin range values will be used as the ranges for the frequencies. Excel will create bin ranges if this is left blank, but the ranges Excel chooses may not provide a useful histogram.

3. **Labels in first row:** Check this box if the data in the input range includes the data labels in the first row. This tells Excel to use the first row as titles and not actual data values.

4. **Output options:** The location options for the output should be presented. In this example, the output will be placed starting in cell E1 of the current worksheet. The output may also be placed in a new worksheet or a new workbook.

5. **Pareto:** Check this box to produce a Pareto chart. A Pareto chart orders the bars in descending order. Pareto charts are not covered in this text.

6. **Cumulative percentage:** The cumulative percentage as well as the frequency within the bins will be reported in the output if this box is checked.

7. **Chart output:** A chart is included in the output in addition to the tabular summary of the bin frequencies.

Figure B.19 | **Histogram output**

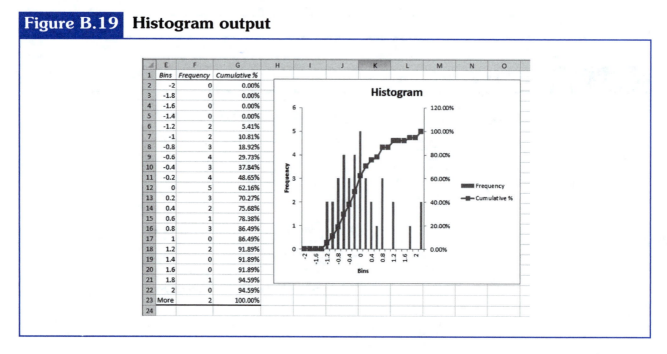

The histogram output for this example shows that the majority of the standardized residuals follow an approximate bell shaped or normal curve. There are some values greater than 0.8 that should be investigated further.

Random Number Generation

The Random Number Generation function was presented in chapter 7 during the discussion of sample selection. The data from example 7.2 will be used to demonstrate the DAT Random Number Generation function. In example 7.2, a sample of 3 subjects is selected at random from the population of 10 subjects.

Select "Data" from the main menu and then click "Data Analysis" on the data ribbon. Figure B.20 shows the Data Analysis menu with "Random Number Generation" selected. Click "OK" after selecting "Random Number Generation."

Figure B.20 **Data analysis window**

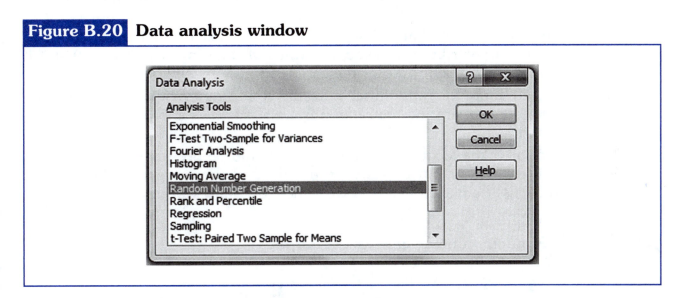

Figure B.21 **Random number generation window**

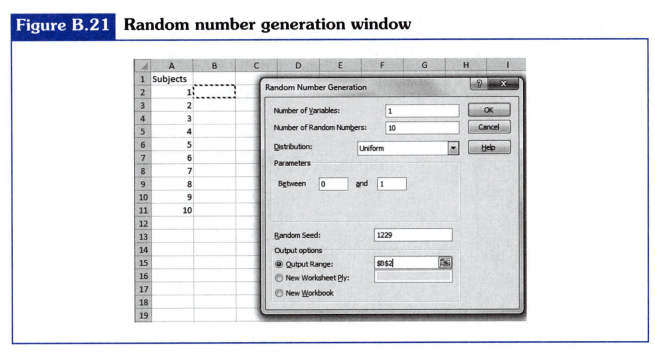

Figure B.21 shows the Random Number Generation window populated for the example data. The data elements required are as follows:

1. Number of variables: The number of columns of random numbers required. Here only one column is needed.

2. Number of random numbers: Determine the number of rows of random numbers required. Each subject needs a random number assigned, so the value is 10 here.

3. Distribution: There are seven choices of distribution here. Uniform is a good choice because it will produce a series of values within a range and allows for the designation of a random seed.

4. Parameters: This value changes depending on the distribution selected above. For the Uniform distribution the default value of the range is between 0 and 1. The default value is fine for most applications.

5. Random seed: Input the random seed. Recall from chapter 7 that setting the random seed before generating the random numbers allows another user to reproduce the series.

6. Output options: The location for the output should be presented. In this example, the output will be placed starting in cell B2 of the current worksheet. The output may also be placed in a new worksheet or a new workbook.

Figure B.22 | **Random number generation output**

	A	B
1	Subjects	Random Numbers
2	1	0.123661
3	2	0.366435743
4	3	0.663624989
5	4	0.595507675
6	5	0.129734184
7	6	0.63637196
8	7	0.991210669
9	8	0.194586016
10	9	0.604327525
11	10	0.344157231

Figure B.22 displays the output for random number generation. The use of the random numbers is outlined in chapter 7.

Regression

Regression was presented in chapter 6 as a statistical tool to model the relationship between two variables. In simple linear regression, one independent variable is used to predict a dependent variable by using a straight line. The slope and intercept of that straight line are estimated using a method called least squares regression. The DAT has a regression function that will be demonstrated using the data from example 6.5. In this example, the independent variable was length of stay. The dependent variable was total charge.

Select "Data" from the main menu and then click "Data Analysis" on the data ribbon. Figure B.23 shows the data analysis menu with "Regression" selected. Click "OK" after selecting "Regression."

Figure B.23 **Data analysis window**

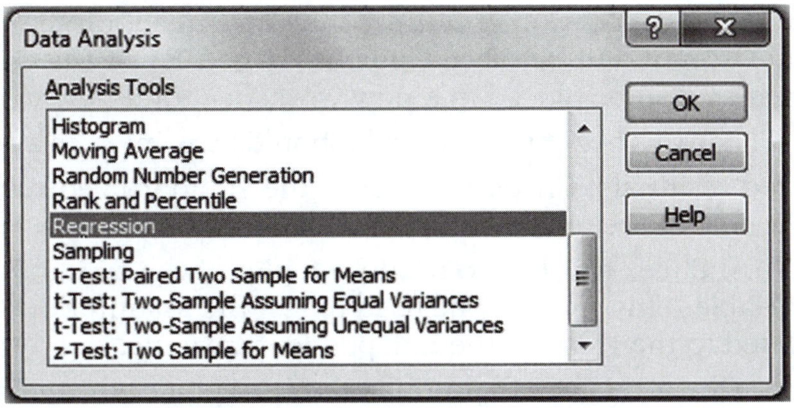

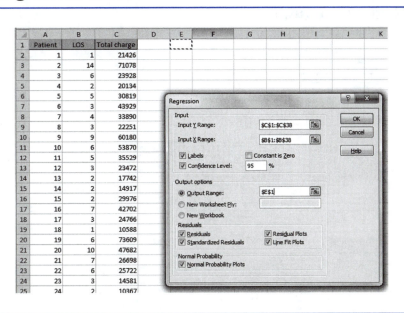

Figure B.24 **Regression window**

Figure B.24 shows the Regression window populated for the example data. The data elements required are as follows:

1. **Input Y range:** The range of values for the dependent variable. Note that the range includes the first row which is the label.

2. **Input X range:** The range of values for the independent variable. Note that the range includes the first row which is the label.

3. **Labels:** Check this box if the first row in the data range is labels. Excel will ignore the labels when calculating the results. Note that the first row of both data ranges will be ignored, so labels should be used in both columns or not at all.

4. **Constant is zero:** Check this box to estimate a regression line with a y-intercept of zero. There are situations where this is appropriate due to the practical application of the model.

5. **Confidence level:** This is the confidence level for confidence intervals for the regression slope and intercept values. If the box is checked, then confidence intervals will be produced for both parameters.

6. **Output options:** The location options for the output should be presented. In this example, the output will be placed starting in cell E1 of the current worksheet. The output may also be placed in a new worksheet or a new workbook.

7. **Residuals:** Check this box if the residuals should be printed as a part of the output.

8. **Standardized residuals:** Check this box if the standardized residuals should be printed as a part of the output.

9. **Residual plots:** Check this box to produce a plot of the residuals versus the independent variable. This plot may be used to test the assumption that the residuals are not related to the value of the independent variable.

10. **Line fit plots:** Check this box to produce a scatter plot of the independent variable versus the dependent variable including the fitted line.

Figure B.25 Regression output

	E	F	G	H	I	J	K	L	M
1	SUMMARY OUTPUT								
2									
3	*Regression Statistics*								
4	Multiple R	0.778577968							
5	R Square	0.606183652							
6	Adjusted R Square	0.594931756							
7	Standard Error	10611.47364							
8	Observations	37							
9									
10	ANOVA								
11		*df*	*SS*	*MS*	*F*	*Significance F*			
12	Regression	1	6066384346	6066384346	53.87391328	1.39897E-08			
13	Residual	35	3941118051	112603372.9					
14	Total	36	10007502397						
15									
16		*Coefficients*	*Standard Error*	*t Stat*	*P-value*	*Lower 95%*	*Upper 95%*	*Lower 95.0%*	*Upper 95.0%*
17	Intercept	9581.934653	3357.02666	2.854292094	0.007200725	2766.808216	16397.06109	2766.808216	16397.06109
18	LOS	4303.427723	586.3072329	7.3398851	1.39897E-08	3113.160761	5493.694685	3113.160761	5493.694685
19									
20									
21									
22	RESIDUAL OUTPUT					PROBABILITY OUTPUT			
23									
24	Observation	Predicted Total charge	Residuals	Standard Residuals		Percentile	Total charge		
25	1	13885.36238	7540.637624	0.720691831		1.351351351	10367		
26	2	69829.92277	1248.077228	0.119284218		4.054054054	10588		
27	3	35402.50099	-11474.50099	-1.096668417		6.756756757	12482		
28	4	18188.7901	1945.209901	0.185912247		9.459459459	14581		
29	5	31099.07327	-280.0732673	-0.026767831		12.16216216	14917		

11. Normal probability: Check this box to produce a plot of the dependent variable versus the normal distribution. If the dependent variable is very different from the normal distribution, then a transformation of the variable may be required. This topic is beyond the scope of this text.

Figure B.25 displays the output for regression excluding the plots. The interpretation of this output is presented in chapter 6.

t-Test: Paired Two-Sample for Means

The t-Test: paired two-sample for means is used to test the hypothesis that there is some difference or change in paired populations. This type of inference was presented in chapter 5. The data for example 5.7 will be used to demonstrate the t-Test: paired two-sample for means function in the DAT. In this example, coder productivity was measured before and after training. The null hypothesis for this test is that the training had no effect or that the pre training mean is equal to the post training mean.

Select "Data" from the main menu and then click "Data Analysis" on the data ribbon. Figure B.26 shows the Data Analysis menu with "t-Test: Paired Two-Sample for Means" selected. Click "OK" after selecting "t-Test: Paired Two-Sample for Means."

Figure B.26 | **Data analysis window**

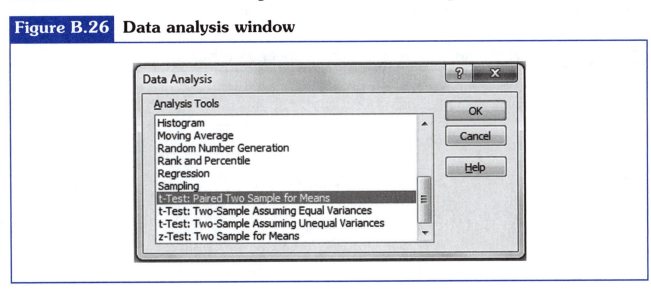

Figure B.27 | **t-Test: paired two-sample for means window**

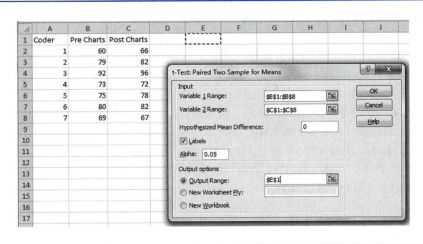

Figure A.27 shows the t-Test: Paired Two Sample for Means window populated for the example. The data elements are as follows:

1. Variable one range: The range for the measurement of the first item in the pair. In this case, B1:B8 represents the pre measurements. Notice that the first row contains the labels for the column of data.

2. Variable two range: The range for the measurement of the second item in the pair. In this case, C1:C8 represents the post measurements. Notice that the first row contains the labels for the column of data.

3. Hypothesized mean difference: In this example, any change is important therefore zero is input here. If a certain level of change is required to be practically significant, then a non zero value may be input here.

4. Labels: Check this box if the first row in the data columns is the title. Excel will ignore this row of data in the analysis.

5. Alpha: The alpha level for the hypothesis test.

6. Output options: The location for the output should be presented. In this example, the output will be placed starting in cell E1 of the current worksheet. The output may also be placed in a new worksheet or a new workbook.

Figure B.28 **t-Test: paired two-sample for means output**

	A	B	C	D	E	F	G
1	Coder	Pre Charts	Post Charts		t-Test: Paired Two Sample for Means		
2	1	60	66				
3	2	79	82			Pre Charts	Post Charts
4	3	92	96		Mean	75.42857143	77.57142857
5	4	73	72		Variance	98.95238095	109.2857143
6	5	75	78		Observations	7	7
7	6	80	82		Pearson Correlation	0.963684366	
8	7	69	67		Hypothesized Mean Difference	0	
9					df	6	
10					t Stat	-2.028756678	
11					P(T<=t) one-tail	0.044408299	
12					t Critical one-tail	1.943180281	
13					P(T<=t) two-tail	0.088816598	
14					t Critical two-tail	2.446911851	

The output of the t-Test: paired two sample for means is presented in figure B.28. The interpretation of this output is discussed in chapter 5.

t-Test: Two-Sample Assuming Equal Variances

The two sample t-test is presented in chapter 5 as a method to determine if the means of two populations are different. The null hypothesis for this test is that the two means are equal and the alternative hypothesis is that the means are unequal. The data from example 5.9 will be used to demonstrate the t-Test: two-sample assuming equal variances function in the DAT. In this example, the mean charges for patients admitted through the emergency department are compared to the mean charges for patients not admitted through the emergency department.

Select "Data" from the main menu and then click "Data Analysis" on the data ribbon. Figure B.26 shows the data analysis menu with "t-Test: two-sample assuming equal variances" selected. Click "OK" after selecting "t-Test: two-sample assuming equal variances."

Figure B.29   Data analysis window

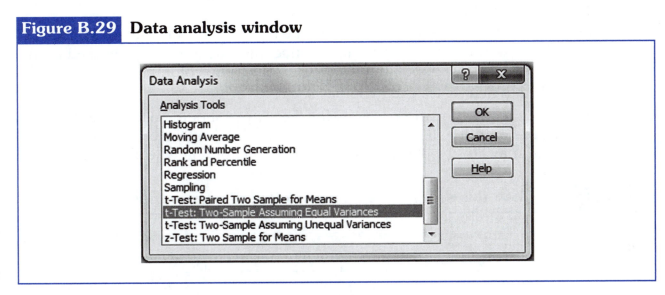

Figure B.30   t-Test: two-sample assuming equal variance window

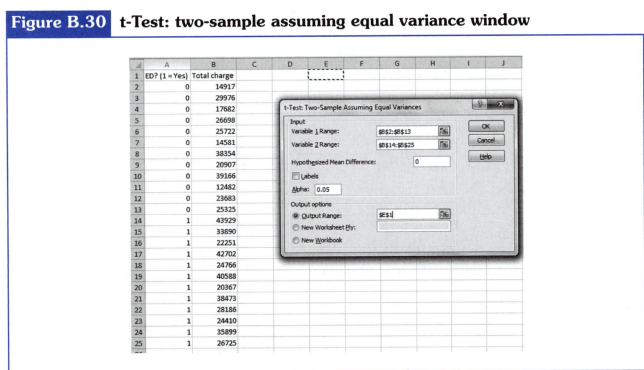

Figure B.30 shows the t-Test: two-sample assuming equal variances window populated for the example. The data elements are as follows:

1. Variable one range: The range for the measurement of the first population: patients not admitted through the emergency department.

2. Variable two range: The range for the measurement of the second population: patients admitted through the emergency department.
3. Hypothesized mean difference: In this example, any difference is important therefore zero is input here. If a certain level of change is required to be practically significant, then a non zero value may be input here.
4. Labels: Check this box if the first row in the data columns is the title. Excel will ignore this row of data in the analysis. Notice that this box is not checked in this example since the two populations appear in the same column.
5. Alpha: The alpha level for the hypothesis test.
6. Output options: The location options for the output should be presented. In this example, the output will be placed starting in cell E1 of the current worksheet. The output may also be placed in a new worksheet or a new workbook.

Figure B.31 t-Test: two-sample assuming equal variances output

	A	B	C	D	E	F	G
1	ED? (1 = Yes)	Total charge			t-Test: Two-Sample Assuming Equal Variances		
2	0	14917					
3	0	29976				*Variable 1*	*Variable 2*
4	0	17682			Mean	24124.41667	31848.83333
5	0	26698			Variance	76094440.27	70333469.97
6	0	25722			Observations	12	12
7	0	14581			Pooled Variance	73213955.12	
8	0	38354			Hypothesized Mean Difference	0	
9	0	20907			df	22	
10	0	39166			t Stat	-2.211283285	
11	0	12482			P(T<=t) one-tail	0.018855962	
12	0	23683			t Critical one-tail	1.717144374	
13	0	25325			P(T<=t) two-tail	0.037711923	
14	1	43929			t Critical two-tail	2.073873068	
15	1	33890					
16	1	22251					
17	1	42702					
18	1	24766					
19	1	40588					
20	1	20367					
21	1	38473					
22	1	28186					
23	1	24410					
24	1	35899					
25	1	26725					

Figure B.31 displays the output of the t-Test: two-sample assuming equal variances function. The interpretation of the output is presented in chapter 5.

t-Test: Two-Sample Assuming Unequal Variances

The two sample t-test is presented in chapter 5 as a method to determine if the means of two populations are different. The null hypothesis for this test is that the two means are equal and the alternative hypothesis is that the means are unequal. In this case, the population variances are unequal and therefore the version of the test for unequal variances must be used. The data from example 5.10 will be used to demonstrate the t-Test: two-sample assuming unequal variances function in the DAT. In this example, the mean length of stay is compared for male and female patients admitted for pneumonia.

Select "Data" from the main menu and then click "Data Analysis" on the data ribbon. Figure B.26 shows the data analysis menu with "t-Test: Two-Sample Assuming Unequal Variances" selected. Click "OK" after selecting "t-Test: Two-Sample Assuming Unequal Variances."

Figure B.32 **Data analysis window**

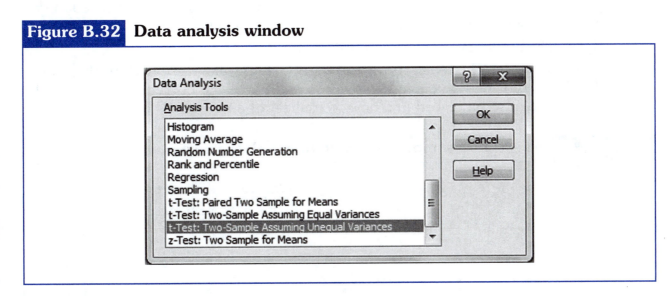

Figure B.33 **t-Test: two-sample assuming unequal variances window**

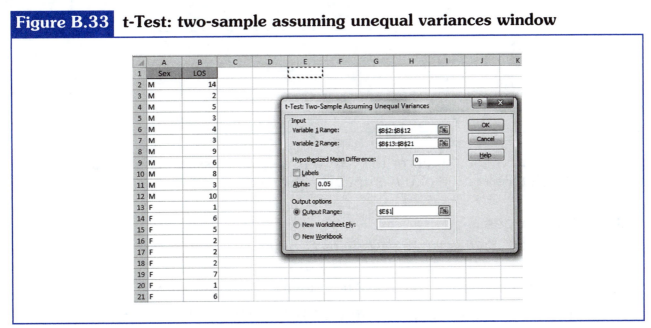

Figure B.33 shows the t-Test: two-sample assuming equal variances window populated for the example. The data elements are as follows:

1. Variable one range: The range for the measurement of the first population: male patients.
2. Variable two range: The range for the measurement of the second population: female patients.

3. Hypothesized mean difference: In this example, any difference is important therefore zero is input here. If a certain level of change is required to be practically significant, then a non zero value may be input here.
4. Labels: Check this box if the first row in the data columns is the title. Excel will ignore this row of data in the analysis. Notice that this box is not checked in this example since the two populations appear in the same column.
5. Alpha: The alpha level for the hypothesis test.
6. Output options: The location for the output should be presented. In this example, the output will be placed starting in cell E1 of the current worksheet. The output may also be placed in a new worksheet or a new workbook.

Figure B.34 t-Test: two-sample assuming unequal variance output

	A	B	C	D	E	F	G
1	Sex	LOS			t-Test: Two-Sample Assuming Unequal Variances		
2	M	14					
3	M	2				*Variable 1*	*Variable 2*
4	M	5			Mean	6.090909091	3.555555556
5	M	3			Variance	14.09090909	5.777777778
6	M	4			Observations	11	9
7	M	3			Hypothesized Mean Difference	0	
8	M	9			df	17	
9	M	6			t Stat	1.828321668	
10	M	8			P(T<=t) one-tail	0.042551696	
11	M	3			t Critical one-tail	1.739606726	
12	M	10			P(T<=t) two-tail	0.085103391	
13	F	1			t Critical two-tail	2.109815578	
14	F	6					
15	F	5					
16	F	2					
17	F	2					
18	F	2					
19	F	7					
20	F	1					
21	F	6					

Figure B.34 displays the output of the t-Test: two-sample assuming unequal variances function. The interpretation of the output is presented in chapter 5.

Other References

Schmuller, J. 2009. *Statistical Analysis with Excel For Dummies, 2nd ed. ISBN: 978-0-470-45406-0*

Links to further explanations of DAT functionality and more examples:

- http://www.bettersolutions.com/excel/EUN147/QP514412778.htm
- http://www.stattutorials.com/EXCEL/index.html

Appendix C: Certified Health Data Analyst (CHDA)

The Certified Health Data Analyst (CHDA) designation was created to meet the demands of the healthcare industry that continues to become more data driven and data dependent.

Individuals who earn the CHDA designation will achieve recognition of their expertise in health data analysis and validation of their mastery of this domain. The pursuit of this prestigious certification will provide practitioners with the knowledge to acquire, manage, analyze, interpret, and transform data into accurate, consistent, and timely information, while balancing the big picture strategic vision with day-to-day details. CHDA-certified professionals will exhibit broad organizational knowledge and the ability to communicate with individuals and groups at multiple levels, both internal and external.

Expanded Eligibility Criteria for CHDA
Effective January 1, 2012

Candidates must meet one of the following eligibility requirements for the Certified Health Data Analyst examination

- Associate's degree and minimum of five (5) years of healthcare data experience
- Healthcare information management credential (RHIT) and minimum of three (3) years of healthcare data experience
- Baccalaureate degree and a minimum of three (3) years of healthcare data experience
- Healthcare information management credential (RHIA) and minimum of one (1) year of healthcare data experience
- Master's or related degree (JD, MD, or PhD) and one (1) year of healthcare data experience

Examination Information

The exam covers the following domains and tasks:

Data Management (32 percent)

Task 1: Assist in the development and maintenance of the data architecture and model to provide a foundation for database design that supports the business' needs.

- Relationship between the data and the organization's strategic goals and priorities
- Data models (conceptual, logical, and physical)
- Basic knowledge of various architecture platforms (Oracle, SQL server)
- Relational database structure (primary key, secondary key)

- Electronic Health Record (EHR) systems
- Database language (SQL, XML)

Task 2: Establish uniform definitions of data captured in source systems to create a reference tool (data dictionary).

- Applicable data standards (ASTM, CDISC, HL7)
- Reference classification/terminology systems and industry data sets requirements (ICD-9-CM, CPT, UB-04, SNOMED, LOINC)

Task 3: Formulate validation strategies and methods (for example, system edits, reports, and audits) to ensure accurate and reliable data.

- Systems testing (integration, load, interface, user acceptance)
- Industry standards (regulatory requirements)
- Best practices for auditing (audit guidelines, system audit trails, and audit logs)

Task 4: Evaluate existing data structures using data tables and field mapping to develop specifications that produce accurate and properly reported data.

- Standard administrative healthcare data (UB-04, CMS form 1500)
- Classification systems data (ICD-9-CM, CPT, SNOMED, LOINC)

Task 5: Integrate data from internal or external sources in order to provide data for analysis and/or reporting.

- Source systems (HIS systems, pharmacy, radiology, financial, etc.)
- Reference classification/terminology systems and industry data sets requirements (ICD-9-CM, CPT, UB-04, SNOMED, LOINC)
- Relational database structure (primary key, secondary key)
- Software applications (word processing, spreadsheet, presentation, and databases)

Task 6: Facilitate the update and maintenance of tables for organizations' information systems in order to ensure the quality and accuracy of the data.

- Applicable data standards (ASTM, CDISC, HL7)
- Source systems (HIS systems, pharmacy, radiology, financial, etc.)
- Reference classification/terminology systems and industry data sets requirements (ICD-9-CM, CPT, UB-04, revenue codes, etc.)
- Classification systems and their history (retirement of codes and their allowed reuse with new descriptors)
- Structure of the data tables
- Scheduled updates of source system content
- Industry standard maps between classification systems

Data Analytics (37 percent)

Task 1: Analyze health data using appropriate testing methods to generate findings for interpretation.

- Basic principles of clinical, financial, and operational data
- Basic understanding of database query syntax (such as SQL)
- Basic understanding of SAS, or SPSS procedures
- Appropriate use of data mining techniques

Task 2: Interpret analytical findings by formulating recommendations for clinical, financial, and operational processes.

- Quality standards, processes, and outcome measures
- Risk adjustment techniques
- Business processes (workflow, system limitations, regulatory and payor guidelines)
- Medical terminology
- Healthcare reimbursement methodologies
- Classification systems
- Industry-standard terms of clinical, financial, and operational data

Task 3: Validate results through qualitative and quantitative analyses to confirm findings.

- Source data content and field attributes
- Qualitative and quantitative analysis techniques
- Healthcare operations to improve clinical and financial outcomes

Data Reporting (31 percent)

Task 1: Design metrics and criteria to meet the end users' needs through the collection and interpretation of data.

- Standard healthcare data sets
- Classification systems and clinical vocabularies and nomenclature (ICD, CPT, HCPC, LOINC, SNOMED-CT, NDC, etc.)
- Basic principles of clinical, financial, and operational data
- Quality standards and outcome measures

Task 2: Generate routine and ad-hoc reports using internal and external data sources to complete data requests.

- Database programs such as Access or SQL Server
- Basic understanding of database query syntax (such as SQL)
- Basic understanding of SAS, or SPSS procedures

Task 3: Present information in a concise, user-friendly format by determining target audience needs to support decision processes.

- Stakeholders within healthcare delivery system
- Software applications (Microsoft Word, Excel, PowerPoint, Access)
- Appropriate modes of presentation (Web conferencing, teleconferencing, AV)

Task 4: Provide recommendations based on analytical results to improve business processes or outcomes.

- Healthcare industry
- Stakeholders within healthcare delivery system

Examination Specifications

The exam lasts for three hours and 45 minutes. All of the questions on the exam are in multiple-choice format.

For additional information and to apply for the exam, visit AHIMA's certification website at www.ahima.org/certification or please contact us by submitting a customer support request at https://secure.ahima.org/contact/contact.aspx or by calling our Customer Relations Team at (800) 335–5535.

AHIMA publishes a variety of study materials for exam preparation. For the most current list of available publications check http://www.ahima.org/publishing. Visit http://www.ahima.org/certification/chda.asp for a list of reference books used by the CHDA Examination Construction Committee to verify the accuracy of the CHDA test questions.

Appendix D: Data Analyst Biographies and Job Descriptions

Data Analyst Biographies

This section contains several biographies of health information management (HIM) professionals who have a career path that includes health data analysis. Each of these biographies shows the different routes the professionals took to their current positions, the differing credentials that each has achieved, and the variety of data types that each works with.

Patience Hoag, RHIT, CHCA, CHDA, CCS, CCS-P, CPHQ is an independent consultant, serving as auditor for HEDIS, Pay for Performance, and Performance Measure Validation activities. Hoag started her health information career in the military, beginning as a file clerk. After her discharge, she continued working in clerical and medical support positions, including a position at the intake facility for the Arizona Department of Corrections. Her supervisor at that time, Deborah Dennis, encouraged her to continue her education and obtain her accredited record technician certification.

Many years and a couple of kids later, Hoag returned to school, graduating as a valedictorian with highest distinction from Phoenix College, where she obtained her associate in applied science in health information technology. After graduation, she worked in long-term care and ambulatory care, then landed a position doing coding training with a large multispecialty group practice. Also during this time, she achieved the certified coding specialist—physician-based (CCS-P) and certified coding specialist (CCS) certifications as well as an additional coding certification, which she no longer renews.

Several years later, Hoag had an opportunity to use her coding expertise in a different area: medical claims review for a third-party billing organization. However, she soon learned that her expertise was lost in the company's bottom line—deny payment whenever possible. After struggling with her conscience regarding this activity, she elected to seek another opportunity, this time as a reimbursement and coding compliance specialist for a medium-sized hospital facility. This opportunity took place during the hospital's conversion to the ambulatory payment classification (APC) system for the outpatient prospective payment system (OPPS) as well as the hospital's management information system conversion and Y2K testing phase. Through these projects, Hoag gained a higher level of expertise in data analytics by reviewing utilization and discharged-not-final-billed reports, DRG frequencies, and abstracting and tracking data for QIO and Joint Commission quality initiatives within the facility. In addition, she became more involved in chargemaster review and communication between departments within the facility.

Hoag's experience working with data collected by the QIO and Joint Commission prompted her interest in data abstraction for quality initiatives, and when an opportunity to work at the QIO presented itself, she jumped at the chance. Initially, she reviewed higher-weighted DRG requests from hospitals for Medicare beneficiaries. A few months later, another opportunity opened up in the company: working on a coding validation project. Soon after the project was complete, Hoag helped the company's HEDIS team with health record review activities. Although she did not know much about HEDIS, she had gained a reputation for being a skilled coder, which proved to be an asset to the team.

After learning more about HEDIS and other performance measure validation activities, Hoag requested to be added to the team to be trained as an auditor. She had previously demonstrated her knowledge of healthcare data, reimbursement methodologies, and quality improvement, and her HIM background was an excellent foundation in that regard. To her delight, she was welcomed on the team, and she enthusiastically embraced this new challenge. The activities related to conducting a HEDIS audit meshed well with her background, involving documentation and reports review, on-site auditing, and post–on-site data and rate review.

Once Hoag had several years of experience under her belt, she sat for the certified HEDIS compliance auditor exam, administered by the National Committee for Quality Assurance (NCQA). Her first bid was unsuccessful (which was hard for this former valedictorian to acknowledge), but she did pass the second time through. The additional experience she obtained during this period helped her understand data quality and integrity as well as analysis. Hoag was also added as a panel member on NCQA's HEDIS Coding Expert Panel, which assists in reviewing codes for the different measure specifications.

In addition to her role as a HEDIS auditor, Hoag participated as a coding resource for encounter data validation activities as well as other healthcare quality projects throughout the year. She also served as a coding expert within the HEDIS audit team, and although she no longer was involved in applying codes on the front end of the data cycle, she tried to keep on top of current issues in the coding world via AHIMA's Communities of Practice tool, as well as by attending continuing education seminars related to coding and healthcare data.

In 2011, Hoag explored opportunities to hone her data analytics and quality improvement skills outside of the QIO. While working as a business consultant for Resolution Health, she was responsible for translating highly complex and varied HIM and coding and reimbursement business needs into application software requirements. During this time, she attained the Certified Professional in Healthcare Quality (CPHQ) credential. In 2012, Hoag worked as Quality Improvement Manager for Coventry Health Care, where she managed organizational quality improvement activities for health services operations. In 2012 Hoag became an AHIMA-Approved ICD-10 CM/ICD-10 PCS trainer, successfully sat for the HITPro Clinician and Practitioner Consultant (EHR Implementation) Exam, and also attained the Certified Health Data Analyst test, a goal she had set for herself years before. Hoag considers herself very fortunate to be in the position she is in because HEDIS auditors typically have a higher level of education than she currently does, and their education is either clinically based or public health-based. While she acknowledges that being at the right place at the right time certainly helped her in her current career path, she feels that if it were not for her background in HIM, along with her proven expertise in coding, she likely would not have been considered a candidate for such a position.

Hoag continues to doggedly pursue her bachelor's degree, which has become a holy grail of sorts—highly desired but very elusive. Her goal is simply to continue to learn and build on the great educational foundation she has achieved in HIM.

Linda Hyde, RHIA, is a consultant specializing in coding and classification systems and health data analytics. Her first exposure to the HIM field came through her mother, who was an ART, and summer jobs in Medical Records at the Henry Ford Hospital in Detroit, MI. This led to enrollment in the HIM program at Indiana University.

After graduation, her first job was as the assistant director of Medical Records at St. Vincent Hospital in Worcester, MA where she eventually became the director. During the 12 years she spent at this 500-bed teaching hospital, Hyde was involved in a number of initiatives that moved the HIM department from manual to computer-supported processes including the development of an in-house abstracting and reporting system. Her last four years at St. Vincent were as the assistant director of the Quality Assurance Division, which included the Medical Record, Utilization and Risk Management, and Medical Staff support departments. Data analytics became a primary focus of her work, both in the development of computer systems to collect data and on the reporting side.

Hyde then became a founding member of a newly formed company, MediQual Systems, to develop a commercial product based on research done in conjunction with St. Vincent on a clinical risk-adjustment methodology to provide severity adjustment for analysis of hospital outcomes. This became the foundation for the risk-adjustment methodology used by Pennsylvania for public reporting of hospital performance from the inception of the program. In 1996, MediQual was acquired by Cardinal Health and ultimately became part of CareFusion.

Hyde has played many different roles during her 28 years at MediQual, first in software development, where she developed requirements and directed the software quality assurance team. Her HIM background was instrumental to insuring that developers understood the needs of the user, the type of data that was being collected, and how to present the data for analysis. Hyde has worked with all types of patient data and her accomplishments have included creating mappings to standardize laboratory and pharmacy data and integrating this with demographic and billing data to create a robust database for analyzing hospital outcomes and processes. In addition, she served as the primary lead in the integration of the data collection and submission for the Joint Commission ORYX program and, ultimately, for the National Hospital Quality Initiatives program for both the Joint Commission and Centers for Medicare and Medicaid Services.

These activities transitioned into other roles, involving project management and directing a team of data analysts as part of a research team supporting maintenance of the risk-adjustment methodology used in the products and services offered by the company as well as in external projects analyzing hospital outcomes and process data for presentation and publication at medical conferences.

Hyde and Karen Derby, a principal data analyst on the team, provided background information on the use of relational databases and statistical software packages for this book.

Hyde is currently using her experience consulting on projects ranging from data mapping and transitioning clinical quality measures for the EHR to standardizing collection of laboratory and pharmacy data for outcomes analysis.

Hyde is an example of how HIM professionals can use their skills to move from a more traditional role into new territory and shows the opportunities for members to serve in many different roles depending on their interest and background.

Grant Landsbach, RHIA, is currently a Data Integrity and EMPI Manager, but was formerly a senior application analyst for Exempla Healthcare in Denver, CO. Landsbach began his HIM career five years ago when he transitioned to healthcare from an information technology (IT) role at an arts organization. He always wanted to be in healthcare and was looking for a way to get into that industry while building upon the IT knowledge and experience he had already gained. After doing some research on health information and different career paths within the healthcare industry, he went back to school at Regis University in Denver, CO. He enrolled in its RHIA certificate program, seeing it as a way to extend his previous bachelor's degree.

Landsbach was hired on with Exempla Healthcare during his first semester in the Regis program and served Exempla in several capacities until he was promoted to his current role. The experience he gained in various roles with Exempla as well as the completion of his RHIA certificate and credential prepared him very well for his current job.

Landsbach's position of senior application analyst is a technical HIM role. Along with his colleagues, he primarily managed the organization's patient information systems. The systems themselves (their hardware and software) and the information contained within them fell within the scope of his job description. The systems he managed contain confidential patient medical information; however, in addition to actual medical information, there are also identification, legal, insurance, and proprietary documents. This information is used by the healthcare organization to treat patients, conduct educational research, relay information to governmental organizations, bill appropriately, and legally document everything that occurs to every patient within the organization. Information contained in the systems must be tracked for release, and documentation of where, when, and to whom it is released must be kept. Note that information has to be released in both identified and deidentified formats depending on its purpose, and all this must be regulated and managed in the systems.

In addition to providing this information for all of these ongoing purposes, Landsbach and his colleagues looked at this information in the aggregate as well as analyze it regularly to provide system enhancements that ultimately result in better systems capable of delivering faster, more accurate, and more secure information to all of Exempla's providers, staff, and patients.

Many of the functions Landsbach performed on a daily basis could be viewed as more IT-based than HIM-based. That being said, it is the mixture of both his IT and HIM skill sets that is important in this position. Being technical is not enough for a role such as his; people with straight IT experience would have the technical skills to manipulate data but would lack the knowledge of the content contained in that data. This knowledge of the data content is truly where Landsbach's RHIA degree supports him in his work.

For example, because information is only good if it is accurate, Landsbach and his colleagues are always looking at ways to validate the information in their systems and make sure that is it correct. To this end, in addition to helping create interfaces to and from the information systems he is involved with, Landsbach spent a great deal of time validating the sent and received information via those interface feeds. These validations are typically done by running one report (typically from the sending or admitting system) against another report (typically generated by the receiving systems that he manages). This validation between two reports is usually done by using a Java-based tool and by importing multiple lists into Microsoft Access and running queries from within that software to check the reports against each other and generate any outliers. These outliers are then researched and corrected by Landsbach and other Exempla Data Integrity employees, and corrections are made as necessary.

In an effort to continue to protect the functionality, speed, and accessibility of the information systems, Landsbach performed ongoing general database and system maintenance on a daily, weekly, and monthly basis. In addition to daily checks for errors and other database indicators, he worked with a database administrator to help streamline the data in the database itself. From a system level, he and his colleagues are the first line of defense in system issues for most of the information applications they support. Based on the daily work they are doing in both the database and the applications themselves, they will typically be the first to notice any application-wide issues. This happens in many ways. One of the more common ways is when a database queue or workflow process becomes backed up. Typically, the application analysts will notice such an event during their daily routines and then will go out to the server to check the given process or processes that correspond to that queue.

There are many other ways that Landsbach can troubleshoot or find problems, and then his job is simply getting everything back online as soon as possible. For example, in addition to using the skills he has, he will often work with other IT employees and the vendor of the given system to resolve the issue, document it, and come up with a future plan to try and prevent it.

Report writing was a significant aspect of Landsbach's job duties. Report writing software is used to provide management reports as well as to create reports that inform him of potential system issues, workflow issues, content issues, and user audits. Landsbach has learned several report writing software suites including Eureka and Crystal and produces all kinds of reports for management using those applications. He also produces statistics for management, which sometimes cannot be produced by the report writing software. In such cases he will often pull information directly from the databases of the information systems by using SQL queries and other proprietary database software to get the needed results. Landsbach's skill sets are critical here, as having the knowledge of the information itself and the purpose for which it is being used is fundamental to creating a great report or compiling the right statistics.

Perhaps the most challenging part of Landsbach's job was the special projects that came along. Many of these projects dealt with antiquated data that either need to be updated to a new and different format or moved into a new system. In many cases, identification numbers and other information will need to be updated or converted in preparation for the new system or storage format. These projects are extremely involved and require a very detailed plan as well as some degree of project management skills.

Landsbach, who is now pursuing his master's degree in computer information systems and is looking at an emphasis in informatics, feels very blessed to have the position he currently holds and to be in healthcare. He feels that he is using his skills to create better, faster, and safer information systems and that he directly contributes to saving lives in the process. He is a strong advocate of the health information field and the adoption of technology in that field to produce the aforementioned results.

Data Analyst Job Descriptions

Sample job descriptions for the data analyst position and the data quality manager were created by AHIMA and are provided here to give a general overview of the types of duties performed for each of these positions. Additional information about the skills required for the data analysts and common job titles can be found in chapter 1.

Data Analyst
Sample Job Description

General Purpose: Provide expertise to acquire, manage, manipulate, and analyze data and report results.

Responsibilities:

Daily Operations

- Identify data problematic areas and conduct research to determine the best course of action
- Analyze and problem solve issues with current and planned systems as they relate to the integration and management of patient data (for example, review for accuracy in record merge, unmerge processes)
- Analyze reports of data duplicates or other errors to provide ongoing, appropriate interdepartmental communication and monthly or daily data reports (for example, related to the EMPI)
- Monitor for timely and accurate completion of select data elements (for example, verbal physician orders)
- Identify, analyze, and interpret trends or patterns in complex datasets
- Monitor data dictionary statistics

Data Capture

- In collaboration with others, develop and maintain databases and data systems necessary for projects and department functions
- Acquire and abstract primary or secondary data from existing internal or external data sources
- In collaboration with others, develop and implement data collection systems and other strategies that optimize statistical efficiency and data quality
- Perform data entry, either manually or using scanning technology, when needed or required

Data Reporting

- In collaboration with others, interpret data and develop recommendations based on findings
- Develop graphs, reports, and presentations of project results
- Perform basic statistical analyses for projects and reports
- Create and present quality dashboards
- Generate routine and ad hoc reports

Knowledge and Skills

- Technical expertise regarding data models and database design development
- Understanding of XML and SQL
- Proficiency in MS Word, Excel, Access, and PowerPoint
- Experience using SAS®, SPSS, or other statistical package is desirable for analyzing large datasets
- Programming skills preferred; adept at queries and report writing
- Knowledge of statistics, at least to the degree necessary in order to communicate easily with statisticians
- Experience in data mining techniques and procedures and knowing when their use is appropriate
- Ability to present complex information in an understandable and compelling manner

Preferred Qualifications

- Bachelor's degree in information management, healthcare information, computing, mathematics, statistics, or related field
- Healthcare background or experience
- Previous data analyst experience

Data Quality Manager
Sample Job Description

General Purpose: The Data Quality Manager is responsible for developing, implementing, and maintaining a data quality management (compliance) plan for coding and reimbursement, health records and documentation, and quality data in all divisions of the organization.

Reports to: Director of Health Information Management

Responsibilities:

Daily Operations

- Implement and maintain a standardized, organization-wide quality data management plan to ensure compliance with external regulatory and accreditation requirements, policies, and procedures, as well as a data integrity pandemic plan and business continuity plan (if applicable)

- Assess data risk, review areas of high risk, investigate identified issues, report data analysis, prevent violations, and take appropriate steps to correct violations

- Assist in identifying and recommending best practices for quality data management

- Promote the adoption of data standards and the creation of standardized minimum and core datasets that support quality data in the health information systems

- Work in collaboration with primary stakeholders to develop data quality methodologies and processes to be applied consistently across information systems for the organization's internal data needs

- Enable maintenance of communication channels to all stakeholders and escalate data quality issues to appropriate stakeholders

- Provide strategic direction, guidance, and leadership to the organization for data integrity

- Provide consulting services in the area of data quality management to individuals, special projects, and departments throughout the organization when appropriate

- Optimize receipt of high-quality data from parent and contract organizations by active participation and leadership in quality monitoring and improvement efforts

- Participate in revenue cycle management and case management as they relate to data quality; partner with the Health Information Management, Finance, Patient Accounts, and Admitting departments to resolve administrative data collection issues and claim denials

- Contribute to the maintenance of the clinical data capture policies and procedures in compliance with standards (for example, the Joint Commission IM measurements) and reporting requirements (for example, the Agency for Healthcare Research and Quality, AHRQ)

Data Monitoring

- Establish, implement, and maintain a formalized data review process for compliance, including a formal review (audit) process and remediation strategies that will support data quality targets

- Develop, implement, validate, and maintain clinical terminologies, a data dictionary, and data models that are used in the information systems; identify and analyze various data mappings and data integrity through data management functions (if applicable)
- Make recommendations to minimize duplication of data sources and ensure there are processes in place to support the collection of quality data in source information systems, moving the organization from reactive data quality management to proactive data quality management
- Develop a data quality reporting tool for Health Record Services; develop other tools that support process standardization
- Perform detailed quality assurance and data mining of the results; troubleshoot gaps, issues, and anomalies, with the ability to direct processes for continuous quality improvement
- In collaboration with stakeholders, identify assessment tools to assist with data profiling for proactive data quality management; recommend business process and technology redesigns that will enhance data integrity

Coding

- In partnership with appropriate personnel, develop and implement standardized, organization-wide coding guidelines and documentation requirements and develop and implement training and educational programs for physicians and coding professionals on an ongoing basis regarding appropriate documentation to support quality coding and data collection
- Establish, implement, and maintain a formalized review process for coding compliance measurement
- Monitor data quality reports for accurate assignment of codes and DRG assignment

Management

- Monitor staff performance and take action as needed to improve performance and for staff development; facilitate lifelong learning
- Develop and maintain a staffing plan and ensure that the staff has the appropriate skill set for the area of responsibility
- Assist department director with annual budget process as it relates to assigned areas; manage budget and provide input to ensure availability of resources and staff

Knowledge, Skills, and Experience

- Experience with clinical classification systems and health information; strong background in medical and facility claims data, ICD-9-CM, DRG, CPT coding, and case mix methodology
- Knowledge of health information systems, database management and design, spreadsheet design, and computer technology

- Strong analytical and problem-solving skills, with experience in the evaluation of data integrity
- Broad knowledge of clinical vocabularies such as SNOMED-CT, LOINC, etc., as they relate to the electronic health record
- Experience with Microsoft Office; proficiency in word processing, spreadsheet, and presentation software
- Knowledge and understanding of networks, hardware, software, and interfaces required to support the magnitude and complexity of data collection
- Basic understanding of SQL and XML concepts; knowledge of data manipulation applications (MS Access, Excel, MS SQL)
- Knowledge of grouper software and chargemaster activities
- Experience with diverse background in several types of settings: acute care, long-term care, post acute care, physician office, etc.
- Experience in project and operational management and knowledge of applied statistics, process analysis, and outcomes analysis

Preferred Qualifications

- 10 years of professional experience, with 5–7 years in clinical, operational, or data quality improvement
- Master's, Bachelor's, or Associate's degree in health information management or a related field
- Supervisory and management experience
- Credentialed as an RHIA or RHIT; CCS preferred

Appendix E: Answers to Odd-Numbered Review Exercises

Chapter 1 Review Exercises

1. c. Calculation of reimbursement for services
3. c. Qualitative
5. c. Exploratory Data Analysis
7. d. All of the above
9. c. Length of stay

Chapter 2 Review Exercises

1. a. Major Diagnostic Categories
3. c. DRG
5. a. Determine payment for physician services
7. a. CMS-1450
9. d. Laboratory values

Chapter 3 Review Exercises

1. a. Interval or ratio
3. c. PROC
5. a. Statistical analysis software package
7. d. Line graph
9. d. SELECT PATIENT_LNAME, PATIENT_FNAME
       FROM PATIENT
       WHERE PHYSICIAN_NAME = 'X'
       AND ENC_YEAR = 2007

Chapter 4 Review Exercises

1. c. CPT codes
3. a. $H_O:p=p_s$ vs $H_A: p \neq p_s$
5. a. The smallest type I error for which the null hypothesis will be rejected

7. a. The null hypothesis would be rejected at the 0.05 level
9. b. Based on the context of the analysis

Chapter 5 Review Exercises

1. c. Mode
3. c. Analysis of Variance
5. c. 4.8
7. b. Average wait time is longer on weekends
9. d. All of the above

Chapter 6 Review Exercises

1. b. Pearson's r
3. d. Spearman's Rho
5. c. 28
7. a. The test statistic increases
9. d. All of the above

Chapter 7 Review Exercises

1. d. Sampling frame
3. b. A sample of the first 10 students entering a classroom
5. c. Cluster sample
7. b. The random numbers will be reproducible
9. b. Estimate the DRG change rate after documentation queries

Chapter 8 Review Exercises

1. b. 2.8893
3. b. Coding and documentation
5. b. Evaluation and management level criteria are reasonable
7. c. Weights assigned to CPT codes to measure resource intensity
9. b. Work RVUs (wRVU)

Chapter 9 Review Exercises

1. d. All of the above
3. a. A graphical display of performance on key metrics
5. c. Physician care
7. c. Leapfrog Group
9. d. Hospital Compare

Alpha level: The level of Type I error that is deemed acceptable based on context in statistical hypothesis testing. *See* Type I error.

Alternative hypothesis: The complement of the null hypothesis that is to be tested using the appropriate statistical test. This hypothesis typically requires some action to be taken.

Ambulatory payment classification (APC): The payment unit used in the hospital outpatient prospective payment system (OPPS). The classification is a resource-based reimbursement system.

Analysis of variance: The statistical tool used to compare more than two population means. The null hypothesis tests that all of the population means are equal.

Analysis: Reviewing and summarizing data for use in decision making.

Auditing: The performance of internal and external reviews (audits) to identify variations from established baselines (for example, review of outpatient coding as compared with CMS outpatient coding guidelines).

Balanced design: An experimental design where the number of subjects in each sample are the same for all populations sampled. The term is relevant when performing an analysis of variance or a two sample t-test.

Bell curve: The shape of the normal distribution. The bell peaks at the average and slopes down on both sides symmetrically.

Binomial variable: A variable that takes only two values (such as yes or no; alive or dead). The probability of a yes or no is constant across all of the subjects, and the outcome of each subject is independent of the others.

Case Mix Index (CMI): The average relative weight of all cases treated at a given facility or by a given physician, which reflects the resource intensity or clinical severity of a specific group in relation to the other groups in the classification system; calculated by dividing the sum of the weights of diagnosis-related groups for patients discharged during a given period by the total number of patients discharged.

Centers for Medicare and Medicaid Services (CMS): The division of the Department of Health and Human Services that is responsible for developing healthcare policy in the United States, for administering the Medicare program and the federal portion of the Medicaid program, and maintaining the procedure portion of the International Classification of Diseases, ninth revision, Clinical Modification (ICD-9-CM) and International Classification of Diseases, tenth revision, Procedure Coding System (ICD-10-PCS); called the Health Care Financing Administration (HCFA) prior to 2001.

Chi squared test: A statistical test that is used to test for relationships between categorical variables. The null hypothesis for this test is that there is no association between the two variables. Represented by the symbol χ^2 (where χ is the Greek letter chi.)

Cluster random sampling: The population is divided into groups before the sample is selected. The groups or clusters must be mutually exclusive and exhaustive. (That is, every unit in the population is assigned to one and only one cluster.) Clusters are then randomly selected to make up the sample. Cluster sampling may be performed as single-stage or two-stage.

CMS-1500: 1. The universal insurance claim form developed and approved by the American Medical Association (AMA) and the Centers for Medicare and Medicaid Services (CMS) that physicians use to bill Medicare, Medicaid, and private insurers for professional services provided 2. A Medicare claim form used to bill third-party payers for provider services, for example, physician office visits.

Coefficient of determination: A statistic that measures the amount of variance in a dependent variable explained by one or more independent variables. If there is one independent variable, then this value is the Pearson Correlation Coefficient squared.

Confidence interval: An interval that is centered at the sample estimate of a population value that may be calculated so that it has a preset probability of containing the population value.

Confidence level: The probability that a confidence interval includes the true value of a population statistic.

Contingency tables: A useful method for displaying the relationship between two categorical variables. Each category is displayed as rows or columns. The cells in the table represent the count of subjects with each category attribute.

Convenience sampling: A sampling technique where the selection of units from the population is based on easy availability and/or accessibility.

Correlation: A statistic that is used to describe the association or relationship between two continuous variables.

Critical value: The value that a test statistic must be larger than to conclude statistical significance. The value is based on the alpha level of the test and the distribution of the test statistic if the null hypothesis is true.

Current Procedural Terminology (CPT): A comprehensive, descriptive list of terms and associated numeric and alphanumeric codes used for reporting diagnostic and therapeutic procedures and other medical services performed by physicians; published and updated annually by the American Medical Association.

Data: The dates, numbers, images, symbols, letters, and words that represent basic facts and observations about people, processes, measurements, and conditions.

Database: A self-describing collection of integrated records. Each record has multiple attributes, and each attribute has one or more values per entry. The database is self-describing because it contains a description of its own structure, and it is integrated because it has a relationship between the data items.

Data dictionary: A descriptive list of the names, definitions, and attributes of data elements to be collected in an information system or database whose purpose is to standardize definitions and ensure consistent use.

Data mining: The process of extracting and analyzing large volumes of data from a database for the purpose of identifying hidden and sometimes subtle relationships or patterns and using those relationships to predict behaviors.

Descriptive statistics: A set of statistical techniques used to describe data such as means, frequency distributions, and standard deviations; statistical information that describes the characteristics of a specific group or a population.

Diagnosis-related group (DRGs): A unit of case-mix classification adopted by the federal government and some other payers as a prospective payment mechanism for hospital inpatients in which diseases are placed into groups because related diseases and treatments tend to consume similar amounts of healthcare resources and incur similar amounts of cost; in the Medicare and Medicaid programs, one of more than 500 diagnostic classifications in which cases demonstrate similar resource consumption and length-of-stay patterns. Under the prospective payment system (PPS), hospitals are paid a set fee for treating patients in a single DRG category, regardless of the actual cost of care for the individual.

Diagnostic data: The data obtained when diagnoses or reasons for visit are coded with a diagnostic classification system.

Distribution: The pattern of values for a variable. The distribution may be characterized by center and spread or frequency of values.

Entity relationship diagram: A specific type of data modeling used in conceptual data modeling and the logical-level modeling of relational databases.

Exploratory data analysis: The use of graphical techniques to identify and explore patterns in data.

Frequency chart: A graphical representation of a frequency distribution. Typically displayed as a bar chart where the height of the bars represent the frequency of observations in each category.

Frequency distribution: A table or graph that displays the number of times (frequency) a particular observation occurs.

Healthcare Common Procedure Coding System (HCPCS): An alphanumeric classification system that identifies healthcare procedures, equipment, and supplies for claim submission purposes; the three levels are as follows: I, Current Procedural Terminology codes, developed by the AMA; II, codes for equipment, supplies, and services not covered by Current Procedural Terminology codes as well as modifiers that can be used with all levels of codes, developed by CMS; and III (eliminated December 31, 2003, to comply with HIPAA), local codes developed by regional Medicare Part B carriers and used to report physicians' services and supplies to Medicare for reimbursement.

Healthcare Effectiveness Data and Information Set (HEDIS): A set of performance measures developed by the National Commission for Quality Assurance that are designed to provide purchasers and consumers of healthcare with the information they need to compare the performance of managed care plans.

Hospital Compare: A CMS-maintained website that reports the values of the quality indicators required for providers to participate in the Medicare value-based purchasing program.

Hypothesis testing: A statistical method that allows an analyst to measure the strength of evidence from the data to reject or not reject a research hypothesis.

Independent: The statistical term for the lack of relationship of two variables.

Inferential statistics: 1. Statistics that are used to make inferences from a smaller group of data to a large one 2. A set of statistical techniques that allows researchers to make generalizations about a population's characteristics (parameters) on the basis of a sample's characteristics.

Inpatient prospective payment system (IPPS): Payment system used by CMS to reimbursed providers for inpatient hospital services provided to Medicare beneficiaries.

Interval scale: Numeric data where the distance between two values has meaning, but multiplying values has no meaning. Interval scale variables have no true zero value. Temperature measurement is an example of interval data.

Judgment sampling: A sampling technique where the researcher relies on his or her own judgment to select the subjects based on relevant expertise.

Least squares regression line: The line that minimizes the sum of the squared error values between the data points and the line. The line should be as close as possible to all points and not above or below all of them, so the value to be minimized is the squared error values to remove the positive or negative sign from the residual.

Levene's test: A hypothesis test used to test the hypothesis that two population variances are equal.

Logical Observation Identifiers Names and Codes (LOINC): A database protocol developed by the Regenstrief Institute for Health Care, aimed at standardizing laboratory and clinical codes for use in clinical care, outcomes management, and research.

Major diagnostic category (MDC): Under diagnosis-related groups (DRGs), one of 25 categories based on single or multiple organ systems into which all diseases and disorders relating to that system are classified.

Margin of error: The half-width of a confidence interval. For example, if the 95 percent confidence interval for a population mean is (2,4), then the half width is 1. A confidence interval may be expressed as the estimate of the center plus or minus the margin of error or 3±1 in this case.

Mean: A measure of central tendency that is determined by calculating the arithmetic average of the observations in a frequency distribution.

Measures of central tendency: The typical or average value that is descriptive of the entire collection of data for a specific population.

Median: A measure of central tendency that shows the midpoint of a frequency distribution when the observations have been arranged in order from lowest to highest.

Mode: A measure of central tendency that consists of the most frequent observation in a frequency distribution.

National Drug Codes (NDC): Codes that serve as product identifiers for human drugs, currently limited to prescription drugs and a few selected over-the-counter products.

Nominal scale: Measurement scale that consists of categories with no natural or inferred order. Examples include: diagnosis codes, clinical units, and color.

Non probability sampling: A sampling methodology where members of a sample are deliberately selected for a specified purpose. The sample is not selected at random and may not be used to make inference about the population.

Null hypothesis: In hypothesis testing, the null hypothesis is typically the status quo or neutral position.

One-sample t-test: A hypothesis test for the sample mean that is used to test if the sample data collected supports the null hypothesis that the population mean is equal to a fixed or standard value.

One sample Z-test for proportions: A hypothesis test for sample proportions that is used to test if the sample data collected supports the null hypothesis that the population proportion is equal to a fixed or standard value.

Ordinal scale: Measurement scale that consists of categories with a natural or inferred order. Examples include patient satisfaction scores, severity scores, and clinic visit level.

Outpatient Prospective Payment System (OPPS): The Medicare prospective payment system used for hospital-based outpatient services and procedures that is predicated on the assignment of ambulatory payment classifications.

P-value: 1. The probability of incorrectly rejecting the null hypothesis given the sample data collected. 2. The smallest alpha level for which the null hypothesis would be rejected.

Paired t-test: A hypothesis test used to compare a variable measured at two time points on the same subject or comparing values between match pairs. The null hypothesis is that there is no difference between the two time point or pair means.

Pearson's r: A statistic that measures the strength of the linear relationship between two continuous variables. The statistic can range from -1 to $+1$.

Percentile rank: Designates the position of an observation in a group based on the percent of the observations less than or equal to that value. For example, if a score is the 54th percentile, that means that 54 percent of the values are lower than that score.

Pie chart: A graphic technique in which the proportions of a category are displayed as portions of a circle (like pieces of a pie); used to show the relationship of individual parts to the whole.

Population: The universe of data under investigation from which a sample is taken.

Predictive modeling: A process used to identify patterns that can be used to predict the odds of a particular outcome based on the observed data.

Primary data analysis: The analysis of original research data by the researchers who collected them.

Primary use: Using data for the purpose it was collected.

Probability sampling: Each member of a population has a known probability of being selected for the sample.

Procedural data: The data obtained when procedures are coded via a procedural coding system.

Qualitative: Analysis of data that describes observations about or by a subject. The data is not naturally numeric and must be categorized prior to summary.

Quantitative: Analysis of data that is naturally numeric.

Query: A statement in SQL that defines the data to be selected or updated.

Quota sampling: A sampling technique where the population is first segmented into mutually exclusive subgroups, just as in stratified sampling, and then judgment is used to select the subjects or units from each segment based on a specified proportion.

R squared: *See* Coefficient of Determination.

Random seed: A preset starting point for a random number generator. Setting and recording the random seed ensures that the sample is reproducible.

Rank: Denotes a value's position in a group relative to other values that have been organized in order of magnitude.

Ratio scale: Number data where zero has an interpretation and the values may be doubled or multiplied by a constant and still have meaning. Examples of ratio data include: currency, length of stay, number of admissions, and age.

Relationship database management system: A database management system in which data are organized and managed as a collection of tables.

Relative value unit (RVU): A number assigned to a procedure that describes its difficulty and expense in relationship to other procedures by assigning weights to such factors as personnel, time, and level of skill.

Remittance advice(RA): An explanation of payments (for example, claim denials) made by third-party payers.

Residual: The error term in a statistical model. In simple linear regression, the residual is the vertical distance from each point to the least squares line.

Revenue code: A three-or four-digit number used to categorize charges on the UB-04 claim or in the 837I electronic file associated with the claim.

Sample: A set of units selected for study that represents a population.

Sampling frame: A listing of all of the subjects in the universe or population eligible to be sampled.

Sampling plan: A document that includes a definition of the population, any inclusion or exclusion criteria, and the sampling methodology.

Secondary use: Using data for a purpose other than that for which it was originally collected. For example, using of billing data to measure the quality of care is a secondary use. The primary use of that data is to trigger a payment for services.

Seed: See Random seed.

Simple linear regression: A statistical technique used to characterize the linear relationship between a dependent variable and one independent variable.

Simple random sampling: The process of selecting units from a population so that each one has exactly the same chance of being included in the sample.

Slope intercept form: A format for expressing a linear relationship as: $Y = BX + A$. In this formula, B represents the slope of the line and A represents the Y-intercept.

Spearman's Rho: A statistic that measures the strength of the linear relationship between two ordinal variables or one ordinal and one continuous variable. The statistic can range from -1 to $+1$.

SPSS: A software system used to perform statistical analysis.

Standard deviation: A measure of variability that describes the deviation from the mean of a frequency distribution in the original units of measurement; the square root of the variance.

Standard error: The standard deviation of a statistic. Typically, it is the sample standard deviation divided by the square root of the sample size.

Standard normal distribution: Normal distribution with a mean of zero and standard deviation of 1. The normal distribution is the basis for the bell curve.

Standardized residuals: Calculated by subtracting the average residual from each residual and dividing by the standard deviation of the residuals.

Statistical Analysis System (SAS): A software system used to perform statistical analysis.

Strata: Subsets or groupings of subjects that are mutually exclusive and exhaustive. Each subject is assigned to one and only one group.

Stratified random sampling: The process of selecting the same percentages of subjects for a study sample as they exist in the subgroups (strata) of the population.

Structured Query Language (SQL): A fourth-generation computer language that includes both DDL and DML components and is used to create and manipulate relational databases.

Systematic random sample: The process of selecting a sample of subjects for a study by drawing every nth unit on a list.

T test for correlations: A test statistic used to test the null hypothesis that the correlation between two variables is zero.

Test statistic: A statistic used to test a statistical hypothesis.

Tukey Honest Significant Difference (HSD) Test: A post-hoc test used to test the statistical significance of the difference between each pair of means after the null hypothesis in an analysis of variance is rejected.

Two-sample t-test: A hypothesis test for sample means that is used to test if the sample data collected supports the null hypothesis that the two population means are equal.

Two-sample Z-test for proportions: A hypothesis test for sample proportions that is used to test if the sample data collected supports the null hypothesis that the two population proportions are equal.

Type I error: A type of error in which the researcher erroneously rejects the null hypothesis when it is true.

Type II error: A type of error in which the researcher erroneously fails to reject the null hypothesis when it is false.

Uniform Bill-04(UB-04): The single standardized Medicare form for standardized uniform billing, implemented in 2007 for hospital inpatients and outpatients; this form will also be used by the major third-party payers and most hospitals.

Universe: The set of all units that are eligible to be sampled.

Unstructured data: Non numeric, human-readable data. Examples include note fields in an EHR, images, and recorded transcripts.

Variable: A characteristic or property that may take on different values.

Variance: A measure of variability that gives the average of the squared deviations from the mean.

Index